The MAGIC of 3A.M.

by

James O. Page

a JEMS book

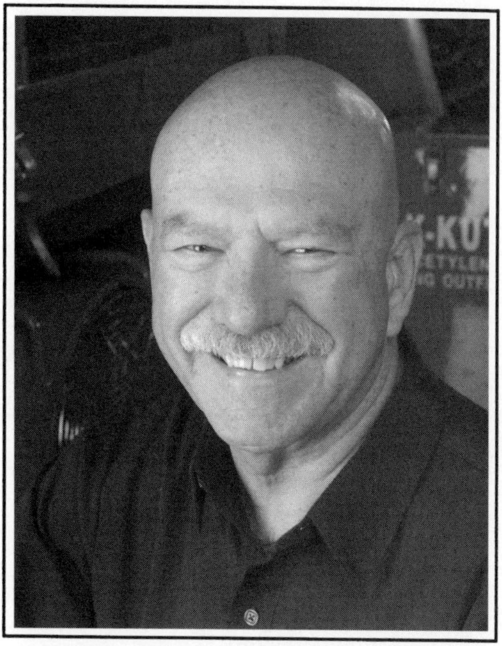

The MAGIC of 3A.M.

Published by:
Jems Communications, JEMS, *Journal of Emergency Medical Services*

Publisher:
Jeff Berend

Cover Design & Production
Janene Long-Forman

ISBN: 0-936174-13-7

JEMS, *Journal of Emergency Medical Services,* is published by:
Jems Communications
1947 Camino Vida Roble, Ste. 200
Carlsbad, CA 92008
760/431-9797 Fax 760/431-8176
www.jems.com

MosbyJems ELSEVIER SCIENCE

Printed and bound in the United States of America.

Cover photo and inside photo by Tom Page

Dedicated to those who give countless hours to training and preparation, who forsake opportunities for wealth, who disregard their own convenience and safety in caring for ill and injured people — quite often at 3 a.m.

Contents

Foreword

The TV series "Emergency!" inspired thousands to become EMTs and paramedics. For thousands more, it was the book *The Magic of 3 a.m.* that inspired them to make EMS their career. The central figure behind both, of course, is James O. Page: fire chief, attorney, state EMS director, "Emergency!" technical adviser, founder and publisher of *JEMS (Journal of Emergency Medical Services)*, prolific author and speaker … the list goes on.

When *Magic* was first published in 1986, it was, in many ways, the anthem for the "Emergency!" generation. This was their story—why they entered the field of EMS, why they continue to care for people in their time of greatest need … often at 3 a.m.

With his typical honesty and clarity, Jim Page's collection of "essays on the art and science of emergency medical services" is not only an entertaining read, but each story is filled with poignant lessons and advice. Simply stated, Jim Page is EMS' finest storyteller. After all, he writes like he talks—as an incredibly gifted orator who's given more than 800 public speeches.

If you think the material might be dated, just take a look at the dedication on page V. Sounds like you, doesn't it? That's why, 16 years after its first printing, the staff of Jems decided to undertake a new printing of *Magic*.

This 2002 edition is for the EMS journeymen and women—the folks who've been there from the start and who are now our nation's EMS leaders. We hope a fresh read of *Magic* will rededicate you to improving EMS and patient care and to training and mentoring the next generation.

It's also for the new generation of EMTs and paramedics—many of whom have only a distant understanding of EMS' tumultuous evolution during the mid-'70s to mid-'80s. These essays will help new EMTs and paramedics have a better understanding of where we've been, which will help them take EMS into the future.

This reprinting of *Magic* also coincides with an important tribute to the life work of James O. Page. A display dedicated to Jim's profound impact on emergency medical services will be inducted into the Julian Stanley Wise/To the Rescue museum in Roanoke, Va., at the same time this book is printed.

You hold in your hands an important part of EMS history—a book that's just as relevant and resonant today as it was 16 years ago, and a book that should be read by everyone involved in EMS.

Jeff Berend
May 2002

Note: For those who would like to learn more about the history of EMS in Jim Page's own words, take a look at the video "Making a Difference: The History of Modern EMS" (available at www.jems.com)

Preface

Everybody's different, but everbody still needs to express himself. For some, it's painting or sculpture. For others, it's sports, or clothing or hairstyle. For as long as I can remember, I've needed to express myself in words — both verbal and written.

Apparently, it was God's will that I should be able to share my thoughts and observations with others. For many years, I've had plenty of access to audiences and readers, and for that I am grateful. To my continual surprise, the audiences and the readers seem to enjoy my personal form of expression.

I've always admired the way painters and photographers look at something and really see it. My artist friends say they appreciate my ability to mold ideas and images into words. Everybody's different but everybody needs to express himself.

A glance through this book will reveal that most of what I write and speak about has something to do with emergencies, medicine, service, and the people on either end of those topics. Those topics and those people have held my attention and stirred my creativity for more than three decades. That should come as no surprise to the men and women who care for others during episodes of great need, fear and desperation. Inexplicably, they are attracted by the opportunity to do for the ill, the injured and the victimized what those people are unable to do for themselves.

People have been rescuing other people for centuries. Only in the last thirty years or so, however, have rescuers begun to react to emergencies with planned precision, some scientific applications, and a systematic use of people and resources. The result of all this change can be measured favorably against the ultimate standards of achievement — lives saved, disability minimized, and suffering reduced. Still, no matter how good the outcome, change is never easy for our species, especially when it flies in the face of comfortable habits and long-standing tradition.

An artist can look at a turbulent sea, capture the image, and re-create the power and the mood of the angry ocean on canvas. It has been my privilege to witness and be a part of the turbulent events which have changed the culture of rescue and emergency medical care. I have tried to capture the images and to re-create them in words. As each word picture is completed, I submit it to the printer and then wait with anxiety for the criticism or acclaim.

When acclaim does occur, I tend to wonder why better writers have not challenged my occupancy of the virgin turf that I write about. The field of emergency medical services is a well-spring of all the things that make for good story-telling and writing — danger, bravery, pain, caring, death, birth, conflict, action, intrigue, excitement, frustration, humor, failure.... Through selection and presentation of words on paper, I have tried to share my impressions in an entertaining format, even though they often deal with the most painful human issues.

Free access to a monthly magazine or to a speaker's podium carries with it some sobering responsibility. Thus, I've always treated with respect the reaction and feedback from readers. Some columns have generated no response while others have primed the pump of reader opinion. Through it all, however, there is a very clear message: People, as a general rule, are pleased to spend time, money and energy to read or hear a message that consists of nothing more than the plain truth and common sense.

It is my sincere hope that you find some plain truth and common sense in this collection of my "art."

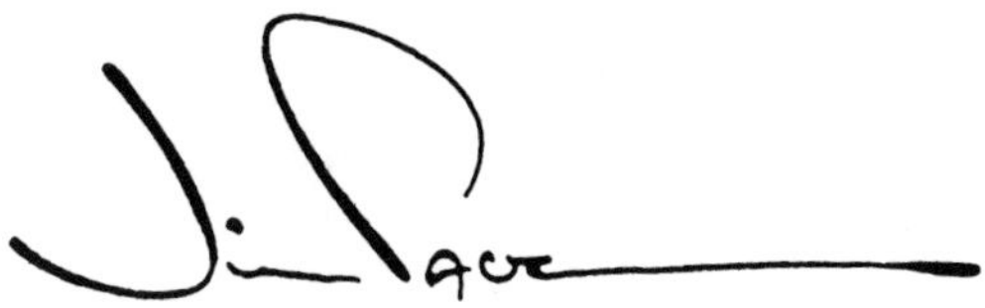

1

The Lure of the Street

Shades of Gray

February 1st was a Saturday. In my little corner of the world, it was sunny and warm. Early in the afternoon, I was running laps at the local high school track. The warm sun was broken by gentle ocean breezes. For some reason, I felt stronger than usual and the track passed beneath me without the usual struggle. I ran for nearly an hour, thanking God at least once each lap for good health, and a bountiful life in a beautiful place.

For awhile, there was another runner on the track. He was about my age and, except for about 20 excess pounds, had the look of an athlete. He would jog a half lap and then walk for a lap or so before jogging again. As I passed him, I thought he seemed to be sweating a lot for that slow pace. As I went around him, I said "Hi." He didn't answer. On the next lap, I noticed he had left.

Twenty-four hours later (Sunday afternoon), I was at my fire department office, cleaning up some random paperwork. Over the radio monitor, I heard an engine company and a rescue ambulance rolling to a near-drowning in one end of the city. A few minutes later, another engine and an ambulance were rolling to an injury report at a shopping mall on the other end of the city. Before I could return attention to my paperwork, I heard the dispatcher report a third medical emergency. There was an uncommon urgency in her voice as she broadcast the report of a man down at the high school track. In the next millisecond, I realized that the nearest units were not available. I jumped from my desk and ran for my staff car, grabbing a jump kit from a reserve pumper while en route. Less than two minutes later, I was at the gate to the high school track.

As I ran the 100 yards from the gate to the scene, I noted that a man was face down on the track. A man was pressing on the victim's back and a woman was watching. The woman gasped as I rolled the stricken man over, exposing bluish skin and open, lifeless eyes." I was on the track with this guy yesterday!" I exclaimed as I recognized the victim.

In a matter of seconds, I gave the male bystander a lesson in CPR. Meantime, I retrieved the oxygen bottle, demand valve and mask. Within three minutes of hearing the dispatcher's first report, my newly trained helper and I were performing effective CPR. At some point in all this, I managed to grab my portable radio and ask for a police officer to assist with CPR. A short time later, I looked up and saw Officer Steve Clary sprinting from the gate. He did a two-point landing at the patient's side and, as the bystander moved out of the way, Steve began picture-perfect compressions.

Over Steve's cadence, the female bystander was explaining to us that the man had fallen right in front of her and her friend as they jogged on the track. She said she sprinted to the gate without stopping and ran across the street to a house where she phoned for help. Altogether, from the time he collapsed until she completed the call, she estimated three minutes had passed.

As I heard this, while the paramedics were arriving at the scene, I noticed that our patient's color was much better and that his pupils had constricted back to normal. About that time, I was relieved by a firefighter who had just arrived on an engine company. I remember thanking God for the opportunity to be where I was, trained and equipped as I was, and able to make an important difference to the stricken man. Every instinct in me was saying, "He's gonna make it."

In the next 20 minutes, I stood with a growing group of spectators and watched some textbook EMS. One of my sons arrived on the scene and I explained to him each of the paramedics' actions. Increasingly, I was jubilant. The medics got him back. As they loaded him for transport, he had a bounding pulse and a good blood pressure, although his spontaneous respirations were sporadic. I turned to my son, fighting back my emotions, and said, "*This* is why I'd rather work in EMS than practice law."

Over the next several days, the elation turned to disappointment and then sorrow. Our patient had suffered serious brain damage and would never regain consciousness. I learned that he was a devoted family man, had been married more than 30 years, and that he and his wife recently had returned from three months in the South Pacific. He had picked up some extra weight and was trying to run it off.

The man died about three weeks after he was stricken. During those weeks, I worried about the emotional and financial price his family was paying for an unsuccessful rescue. A lot of ethical questions crossed my mind during those days and nights. Then, a few nights before the man died, I talked to his son by telephone. Though his father would never again be conscious, the son said, "Thank God, it happened where people could help him."

Over the next several days, I thought of that statement many times. I was reminded that every death in the family has more than one victim. In our eyes, what we did for the father was not successful. But success may be something very different for a grieving wife or son; they need to know that everything that could have been done *was* done. In the "game" of saving lives, there are some shades of gray between winning and losing.

It's Not That Simple

A few weeks ago, I attended a tape critique at a hospital. It's a weekly event where tapes of some of the more interesting or challenging cases are played. In attendance were paramedics from three agencies. They were guided through the process by a nurse and an emergency physician. At the end of each tape there is a discussion — covering strengths and weaknesses, some extra medical dimensions to the case, and the patient's outcome.

For those of us who've climbed the career ladder and don't touch sick people anymore, tape critiques are a valuable contact with reality. The process is a necessary reminder of what this business is all about — quick decisions, agile hands, good instincts, lots of knowledge, fate, and taking chances.

One of the tapes reviewed that day had all the elements. The case happened on a busy afternoon and both of the agency's paramedic units were working calls — at opposite ends of their response area. One of the crews was with an elderly woman; they were waiting for a BLS ambulance to transport her to the hospital. Over the radio the medics heard the other crew go available. Immediately the dispatcher assigned the other crew to a call involving a possible drowning — a three-year-old child. It would be a 10- or 12-minute response.

The medics who were waiting with the elderly woman recognized the address. It was about two minutes from their location. They made a quick decision, left their patient at the scene and took off for the drowning case. As the tape revealed, the next 30 minutes enveloped the paramedic team in more human drama than any filmmaker or author could ever describe.

The child had been submersed in a bathtub for an estimated four minutes. On arrival, the medics found a family member performing mouth-to-mouth respirations but there had been no chest compressions. The first ECG reading showed a flat line. Undeterred, the medics notified the hospital they were working a pediatric code and asked for the necessary orders.

Listening to the tape — the self-assured, rapid-fire voice of a paramedic as he and his partner struggled to restore life to the drowned child — a wonderful irony came to mind. We continually write and rewrite protocols, policies, guidelines, rules and regulations, presumably to make sure that the patient will be properly cared for. But in the end, when a little kid's life is ebbing away on the floor of a narrow hallway, with grieving parents and neighbors looking on, everything depends on the hands and minds and guts of the paramedics.

In lectures all across the country I've warned EMTs and paramedics of the legal hazards of "abandoning" patients. Clearly, leaving a patient before that patient is in the hands of some other qualified provider seems to be the cause of numerous lawsuits against EMT and paramedic agencies. In response to the problem, I've offered my own guidelines for avoiding the problem. It all seems so simple.

But I now realize it isn't all that simple after all. There is no such thing as a guideline for all occasions. Furthermore, if our guidelines place undue emphasis on the legal risks, what happens when medics follow the guidelines to the detriment of a patient? My recent encounter with a tape — and the medics whose exceptional performance was recorded on that tape — was a needed reminder that we are in the people business.

In the process of trying to keep everybody's rear covered, we tend to forget that the exceptional performers in EMS occasionally need the liberty to do what they do best — make quick decisions and stick their necks out to save a patient. The effort to make everything and everyone in our society safe and predictable has a certain appeal. On the other hand, some young paramedics recently proved to me that there will always be a need for people who are brave enough to think for themselves and take a chance when a human life is at stake.

The three-year-old child, by the way, is doing well. It looks like he'll have a chance to grow up and live a normal life.

Stress and Strain

Last night, after a long run and a light dinner, I returned to the office and my frequent companion — the word processor. The goal was to grind out a speech I was expected to deliver on the topic of paramedic burnout. But the words did not come. Not the right words, anyway. After committing several paragraphs to the green screen of the CRT, I pushed the "erase" button and went home.

Among the distractions was a trip into New York City scheduled for the next morning. I was to perform as narrator in a video production, and getting a good night's sleep before exposing myself to the camera seemed logical. But, before retiring, I flipped on the TV to find out whether the world was still intact. Lo and behold, there was Telly Savalas playing a lawyer in a TV movie. I'm a sucker for bald heads and lawyer movies. It was a short sleep.

At 6:30 this morning, I was at the Basking Ridge station, waiting for the train into Hoboken. The Erie Lackawanna trains are older than I am, but they're always on time. Also waiting were several other men; they looked sharp in their Brooks Brothers suits and they were reading the *Wall Street Journal*. Stock brokers and mortgage bankers I presumed.

It had rained the night before and the morning air was thick and sticky. The train conductor had left the doors open to move some air through the cars. After a few miles, it was clear that dirt and grit from the tracks was also in the air. At every stop, more Brooks Brothers suits and *Wall Street Journals* came aboard. Several of my fellow travelers caught me gawking at them. They didn't know it, but I was comparing their working life to that of an urban paramedic.

Midway to Hoboken, the pastoral greenery gave way to the grimy reality of decaying cities. The heavy fragrance of wet grass and trees was replaced by the acrid smell of chemicals, refineries, and traffic fumes. The train lurched, pitched, and squealed as our tracks joined and crossed other tracks. Through it all, my fellow travelers kept their noses buried in their newspapers.

We finally arrived at the Hoboken station and I joined the herd of thousands streaming toward the steps that would take us underground to a subway station. The train under the Hudson River from Hoboken to New York only costs 30 cents. If you don't have the correct change, there is a change machine. This morning, it was broken. By the time I had secured change, gone through the turnstile, and crammed myself into the only remaining space on the departing train, I realized I was on the wrong train. Too late.

I ended up beneath the World Trade Center, rather than 6th Avenue and 42nd Street. Again, I joined the herd as it inched its way to the escalators leading to the street.

After several cabs ignored me, I attracted a creaky Checker, climbed in and instructed the driver to take me to 35 West 39th Street. The driver (who had learned to speak and drive in some faraway place) treated me to an adventure that should be franchised by Disneyland.

Arriving at 39th Street, the cab halted in the middle of a crosswalk just as the light changed. Several hundred pedestrians were forced to walk around the cab, and all were giving me the dirty looks that belonged to the driver. After joining still another herd, I arrived at my destination. There, after my 90 minutes of stress and emotional assault, I was treated to a smile and the morning's first cup of coffee.

The filming went smoothly, but lasted most of the day. Then it was time to get back to my tranquil environs. Finally, as the sun was setting in the west, I completed the adventure as the train deposited me in Basking Ridge.

Again, tonight, the word processor is my companion. Again, I'm trying to write about the stresses and strains of being a paramedic. And all I can think about are those millions of poor souls who spend two, or three, or more hours of every working day just getting there and back on dirty, worn-out conveyances, pressed belly to buttocks with the world's greatest variety of strangers. They are subjected to rudeness and hostility, filth and grime, fear, anxiety and confusion — and that's before they even get to their offices or jobs.

Now, where was I? Oh, yes. Paramedic burnout.

The Short Career

"Get yourself a civil service job," my father would say when the subject of a career came up. "At least, you'll have a regular paycheck if we go through another depression." Like many of his generation, he had grown up in abject poverty, his education was limited by the need to go to work at an early age, and he'd suffered many of the consequences of the Great Depression. He wanted a better life for his children and his advice was a mix of his experience and his hopes.

The experience and hopes of my father's generation affected our society in many ways. Social Security, Basic Educational Opportunity Grants, and public and private pension programs are but a few of the examples. In essence, they wanted us to have the opportunity to train for a single occupation or profession, to spend our working lives at it without concern for lay-offs, and to eventually retire with a comfortable guaranteed income. It's one version of the American Dream.

Ever since EMS emerged as a possible career, we've been hearing about career "burnout" of EMS personnel and some indefinite concepts of a "career ladder" as a cure for the problem. In 1980, *JEMS* took a hard look at one such proposal to provide a career ladder within an EMS system. In the end, costs for operating the system would have risen more than 1,000 percent and only three percent of the workers would have had the opportunity to climb the ladder.

Much has changed since my father's generation influenced our opportunities for education, career and retirement. Many college graduates have found that their chosen careers have no vacancies and that they are "overqualified" for most other jobs. Even federal employees have found that the security of their jobs can erode under a wave of "RIF" notices (reduction in force). Surely one of the greatest American tragedies is the life-long employee who learns too late that his pension system will not provide the income or security he had been counting on.

It would be easy to read these changes — this evaporation of what we have come to know as "security" — in a negative or depressing light. But we should remember that crisis often equals opportunity. In many ways, we have the opportunity to escape from the one-dimensional (and often unsatisfying) career patterns that were thankfully indulged by my father's generation. Their most vivid memories included escaping the dustbowl with the family's entire possessions tied onto an old Ford. They remembered having no shoes, and holes in their only pair of pants. They remembered destitute old folks surviving on the generosity of their destitute children. In their prayers, my father's generation would give thanks for having *any* job — it didn't matter that it was hot, dirty, boring, one-dimensional or unsatisfying.

Regardless of their efforts to create a better life for us, it appears that our working life is what *we* make it. There is no real security. Our master plan for a career can be overturned by international events, a downturn in the economy, a crazy or incompetent boss, or health problems. Given that fact, why do we insist on pursuing a single lifelong career? Why don't we make the most of our working years by changing careers every decade or so? When we reach a dead end in one career, why not make a conscious and intelligent decision to strike out in another career with new challenges and new opportunities?

Which brings me back to EMS as a career. Is it possible that people from my father's generation have created the impression that EMTs and paramedics are supposed to spend their working lives as EMTs and paramedics (with a few getting promoted to supervisory positions)? Is it possible that street medicine is a young person's business — something you do in your prime and then move on to another career? Is it possible that EMT and paramedic attrition and turnover are a part of the business, to be expected, to be planned and budgeted for? Are we simply witnessing a generational change in the whole concept of careers?

Raising the topic of mid-life career changes would have made my father nervous. But without the standard of living that he and his generation created for us, we wouldn't have the liberty to think about much more than survival. Next career, please.

Who's in Charge?

The problem tends to occur at the worst of times. An accident, or a violent crime, or some sort of calamity has placed one or more lives in jeopardy. The call for help brings police officers, firefighters and emergency medical services personnel to the scene. All of them have sworn (or affirmed) their allegiance to some kind of oath which places service to people above all else.

The situation will be made tense by its very nature. The tension may be elevated by a gathering crowd of spectators. Questions will be racing through the minds of the individuals who must care for the victims, preserve evidence, control the crowds, prevent or combat fire, or keep the traffic moving. Each will have much to think about and the early minutes of the emergency will hit them with an overload of sensory stimuli. The situation will be ripe for losing perspective.

"*Hey Chief, get some water on that gasoline spill*," the young EMT shouted to the older fire chief. The chief's angry response was immediate, loud and disruptive.

"*Move that ambulance outta the traffic lane*," the highway patrolman demanded of the EMTs as they conducted their assessment of an ambulance victim. The rude demand produced a surge of adrenalin in the EMTs. Their attention was diverted from the patient, and their methodical check of the injured person suddenly turned haphazard.

"*Load that guy up and git goin' to the hospital*," shouted the fire captain to the private ambulance paramedic. An evasive vein suddenly became more evasive as the paramedic tensed up in reaction to the captain's order.

Nearly everyone with a year or more of EMS experience has a story to tell about confrontations with other members of the "team." Yet nobody can report a clear victory, one in which the patient benefits.

In 1976, the Michigan Legislature tried to do something about the problem by setting up a structure of authority which would govern care for the patient and control of the scene. The law produced bizzare images of police officers, firefighters, EMTs and paramedics standing over a patient and comparing credentials to see who was entitled to be in charge. Numerous reports from Michigan suggest that the law was a dismal failure. Meanwhile, there have been efforts to copy it in other states.

What is the answer? It may have been stated most clearly by Canadian Police Officer Bob Ciupa: "Any time an interaction between professions occurs which requires a sharing of responsibility and a mingling of professional skills, cooperation can be increased if each side has an understanding of the others' point of view."

About the time we were reading Constable Bob Ciupa's comments for the first time, we came across an item in a West Coast fire service magazine. The caption under a photo said, "EMT-trained California Highway Patrol officers are a great help in these remote accidents." Three years ago, the caption would have read much differently. Since then, however, paramedics have spent some time on orientation tours of duty with highway patrolmen. Highway patrolmen have spent some time riding as observers on mobile intensive care units. At the same time, the primitive first aid training of the patrolman has been upgraded to the level of Emergency Medical Technician.

Cooperation can be increased if each side has an understanding of the others' point of view. Surely, it's been said before. But in the heat and emotion of a life-threatening emergency, those primitive substances ooze from our vital organs and prepare us for fight or flight. In far too many cases, the fight has been with fellow trustees of the public interest. In every case, the person whose life is threatened becomes the real loser.

What can you do to solve or prevent role combat among emergency services personnel in your community? If you are a manager or administrator, you might consider making the first move toward creating better understanding of the others' point of view. Call your counterparts in the other services, invite them to lunch or schedule a meeting. For starters, you might propose a ride-along program. Or you might schedule some joint training sessions on the subject of patient assessment, stabilization and transport. It may not work in every case. But it sure beats 200 politicians trying to devise a law which would require emergency services personnel to apply simple common sense.

Fireman, Save My Child

"Firefighters should fight fires," it has been said. Most often in recent years, that statement has been offered to suggest that firefighters already have an important job to do, and that they should leave emergency medical care and transportation to others.

The proposition nearly achieved the status of official government policy in 1980. In that year, a study group was commissioned by the U.S. Department of Transportation (DOT) to evaluate the concept of "third service" prehospital emergency medical services. That is, public agencies of local government (separate and distinct from fire or police departments) that would have prehospital EMS as their sole function. Third service EMS agencies already exist in Austin, Pittsburgh, Wichita, Cleveland, San Francisco and other locales.

Many suspected that the study group and its federal sponsor undertook their job with a built-in bias against fire service EMS. The U.S. Fire Administration was constructing an ambitious program of support and assistance to fire department EMS programs (subsequently abandoned for the most part) and it looked like a battle between federal agencies was shaping up for dominance in EMS.

In the end, the DOT's "evaluation" of third service EMS did little more than bind the fire service together, albeit temporarily. It also raised questions about why the fire service is involved in EMS. The answers to many of these questions are rooted in 50 or more years of history.

Probably the deepest of these roots feeds from the image of the firefighter as a brave and resourceful person who can extract people from grave danger. An early-American lithograph captured the mental image with a graphic representation of a firefighter carrying a child from a fire. "Fireman, Save My Child," was the title of the piece and its publication over many decades reinforced the image and the expectation.

The array of dangerous situations people get themselves into is limitless. Traditionally, however, there has been one source of help when the situation appears helpless. Call the fire department. Whether it's a fire, a cave-in or collapsed building, a kid swept away in a raging river or a cat in a tree, the public is conditioned to call the fire department.

The evolution of fire departments into prehospital emergency care probably parallels the evolution of medicine itself. Until about 50 years ago, people were fatalistic about medical emergencies. It was considered fate, or "God's will," if one's breathing were to stop suddenly — whether in a hospital or on the street. Physicians themselves could do little in such an event. It didn't occur to people that deadly natural events would someday be reversible in a hospital, much less in a home or public setting.

Hope springs eternal, however, and the early experience of the Columbus (Ohio) Fire Department illustrates how hope may have played a role in the fire service's evolution into EMS. In Columbus, as elsewhere, firefighters once were judged by their ability to "eat smoke." Before the advent of self-contained breathing apparatus, firefighters would race into acrid smoke searching for victims. Those who could tolerate the poisonous gases longest achieved dubious status among their peers and spectators.

As expected, some firefighters were overcome by the smoke and became victims themselves. Numerous inventors came forth with solutions to this problem, including a primitive device known as the "Pulmotor." In 1931, a Pulmotor was donated to the Columbus Fire Department to assist firefighters who had eaten too much smoke. Soon, spectators watched with amazement as the device seemingly brought unconscious firefighters back from near-death.

It was an event in 1934, however, that cast the future of the Columbus department. A lineman was electrocuted on a pole and someone called the fire department. The fire chief and two firefighters arrived with the Pulmotor. They were unable to save the lineman but the newspapers reported their efforts in great detail. Soon, Columbus citizens were calling their fire department for assistance in medical emergencies.

Later that year, a Columbus Fire Department hose wagon was equipped with an H&H Inhalator and supplies donated by the Red Cross. The vehicle was placed in service to respond to calls from the public. In doing so, Columbus joined a handful of fire departments throughout the country that had expanded their traditional fire protection role to include medical rescue and first aid.

Except for some accidents of history more than 50 years ago, Columbus might have been like Cleveland or Tulsa or Pittsburgh. Without the donation of the Pulmotor, without the publicized rescue of the lineman, without an aggressive chief who wanted to expand the department's services to the public, the Columbus Fire Department might have presumed that medical emergencies were someone else's business.

Instead, Columbus' "Number One Inhalator" gained support of citizens and the medical community over the years. As the calls for medical assistance increased, more medical rescue units were placed in service and more firefighters formed competitive first-aid teams. They've won dozens of international awards in rescue and medical care competitions. In Columbus and other departments with two or more generations in medical rescue, it would be difficult to imagine a single-function fire department, limited only to fire protection services.

The accidents of history continued. Dr. James V. Warren was chairman of the department of medicine at Ohio State University in Columbus. He was friendly with Dr. J. Frank Pantridge of Belfast, Northern Ireland. Dr. Pantridge had experimented with mobile coronary care — a system whereby medical and nursing personnel would drive from the hospital to remote locations to treat heart attack victims. At about the same time, Dr. Warren was researching the possibility of mobile coronary care in Columbus.

Using grant monies, the Columbus "Heartmobile" went into service in 1969, staffed on each shift by one cardiologist and three off-duty Columbus Fire Department rescue squad members. Though the program was successful, grants don't last forever. Staffing the mobile coronary care units with doctors would not be possible without the grant funds which were scheduled to end in 1971. Everybody involved with the project had been impressed by the performance of the firefighters, however, and a decision was made to train them to replace the physicians.

In July 1971, the Columbus experiment took a new name and a new shape. The Columbus Fire Department, 40 years after it had been donated a Pulmotor, became one of the first fire departments in the U.S. to provide advanced life support with firefighter paramedics.

At about this time, unknown to the American fire services, its future was being shaped at annual medical meetings. At those meetings, Dr. Warren would meet with colleagues who had been conducting their own experiments with mobile coronary care. Dr. Eugene Nagel had trained some firefighters as paramedics in Miami. Dr. Leonard Cobb had launched the famous "Medic 1" project in cooperation with the Seattle Fire Department. Dr. J. Michael Criley was training firefighters to be paramedics in Los Angeles while Dr. Walter Graf was training firefighters and private ambulance personnel in nearby Inglewood.

Not all the budding advanced life support projects were fire department based. In San Francisco, Dr. Herman Uhley was training private ambulance personnel, as was Dr. Leonard Rose in Portland, Oregon. In a short-lived program in Newark, Dr. Mortimer Schwartz tried to use hospital-based medical personnel to deliver ALS in the field. At St. Vincent's Hospital in New York City, Dr. William Grace launched a program that first used physicians on an ambulance vehicle and later switched to hospital-based paramedics. Dr. Richard Crampton was training volunteer rescue personnel in rural Virginia.

In the early years, though, it was the fire department

programs that proved least expensive and most durable. Most of the fire department paramedic programs were created with existing personnel; no increases in personnel rosters or salary budgets were necessary. The firefighter paramedics were linked to their jobs by stable organizations and pension systems. Attrition of newly trained paramedics in the private ambulance and hospital-based systems was severe.

The pioneering cardiologists presented papers about the new ALS programs at the medical conferences. Other doctors, hearing of these successes in prehospital emergency medical care, went home from the meetings to visit their local fire chiefs. The future of the fire service was being cast from outside.

In many cases, the choice of firefighters as paramedic trainees was based largely on their availability. In the early stages of the Los Angeles program, for example, fire departments simply detailed personnel to paramedic training without budgeting for replacement personnel. In essence, the fire departments were willing to upgrade their existing rescue services with little or no costs borne by the physicians who wanted to experiment with the concept of prehospital advanced life support.

It wasn't the first time that fire departments had been tapped by the medical community. Prior to 1941, many hospitals operated their own ambulances, often staffed with doctors. But the manpower demands of the war forced a transfer of many functions. Fire and police departments in many cities stepped in to take over ambulance service. In other places, private ambulance companies were created to fill the void as hospitals stopped providing the service.

But the historical accidents of the early 1970s had no rivals for their impact on public expectations and the fire service. One such event was the creation of the popular television series, "Emergency!" Based on the Los Angeles County Fire Department's paramedic service, the program broadcast for six seasons and reruns still are shown throughout North America and many foreign countries.

Coinciding with the federal government's major EMS initiative, this weekly television program made emergency medical care (and the fire service) a topic of household conversation throughout the nation. An entire generation of six-year-olds insisted on watching "Emergency!" before going to bed on Saturday nights. This year, those children will be eligible to vote, and old enough to apply for the job of their childhood dreams — a firefighter paramedic.

A 1981 survey covering both career and volunteer fire departments disclosed that 72 percent were providing some form of emergency medical service. It was clear, however, that the approaches to fire service EMS presented by the pioneering paramedic programs and the television series had not been followed everywhere. Only 17 percent of those departments reporting (23.6 percent of departments providing EMS) were trained and operating at the advanced life support level.

Today, many departments simply provide engine company first response, usually in cooperation with another agency or a private ambulance company. At the other end of the scale are those fire departments providing ambulance transportation with advanced life support services. In 1981, 79 percent of all fire department EMS programs were using dual-role, cross-trained personnel.

Despite this national proliferation of fire service involvement in EMS, there remain those — both inside and outside the fire service — who feel that "firefighters should fight fires." We can only speculate on what the fire service would be like today without the public and budgetary support it has reaped from its EMS role. Could a single-function fire service have endured the economic pressures of two oil shortages, double-digit inflation, taxpayer rebellions and the longest of postwar recessions?

But for a few historical accidents, matters might have been much different. What if the private ambulance industry had been better managed in its early years? What if Doctors Warren, Nagel, Cobb and Criley had found the money to create hospital-based paramedic programs? What if NBC had turned down Jack Webb's idea for a television series?

When the final chapter of the fire service EMS story is written, serendipity surely will be recognized as a key factor in the formative years. In the years ahead, on the other hand, it's not likely that there will be the opportunity for things to just happen. In both fire service and health care in a nation flirting with bankruptcy, decisions will be based on cold-eyed analyses of quality and cost. Will the fire service be able to maintain its role in EMS in that environment?

Provided our nation remains a democracy, there may be another factor. The voting public doesn't always conform to the conclusions of the analysts. In the past, the typical citizen harbored the image of the firefighter as the brave and resourceful person who can extract people from grave danger: "Fireman, Save My Child." Unless the fire service abuses or destroys that image, unless some other category of EMS worker displaces that image in the public mind, the public is likely to opt for the familiar image.

Re-enlisting as an EMT

As I write this, I'm in the middle of one of the most difficult but satisfying experiences of my career — a basic EMT course. The difficult part was admitting to myself and others that I had forgotten most of what I had ever known about basic emergency care. Once that barrier was crossed, I signed up, and since then most of my spare time has been devoted to reading, studying and practicing.

Fortunately, most of my fellow students don't know what I do for a living. The course coordinator agreed not to blow my cover. I wanted to go through the course as a typical student would, and I didn't want the additional pressure of having to perform as an expert throughout the course. It had been years since my certification lapsed, and I couldn't have pretended to be an expert anyway.

One of the biggest challenges has been to keep my mouth shut — especially during the medical-legal lecture. The course coordinator and instructors have been superb; they are good at what they do and they really want their students to be skilled EMTs. Thus far, the physician lecturers have done an admirable job.

My attitude about the course really changed when I took the first practice exam. I passed the written but got rattled when the instructor threw an unexpected (but realistic) deviation at me during the CPR practical. "If you can't handle a surprise on a manikin, you won't be able to handle it on a real patient," he said sternly. Of course, he was right. Of course, I was humiliated.

Because of my travel schedule, I've had to miss several classes and attend make-up sessions at a number of locations. The make-up classes have given me an opportunity to observe the differences between courses which are teaching the same basic material. It seems to me that some coordinators and instructors have a greater aptitude for conveying knowledge and skills than do others. It shows in their students, and I presume it will show on the street eventually.

For more than a decade, I have lived and breathed EMS. Virtually everything of significance that's written about emergency care crosses my desk and I read it all. I've seen EMS systems and I've visited with EMS people in 49 states. But not until I decided to re-enlist as an EMT did I realize how much I had forgotten about patient care, and how little I had known in the first place.

At this point, I'm plenty worried about the final exam. But I'm scared by those who feel they don't need EMT training, or who feel that 81 hours of training will serve them for a lifetime. If I ever get through this course, I'm going to pull all those dusty books off the shelf and start rebuilding my rusty base of knowledge. And I'm going to wonder about those who never touch a book after they've sewn on their EMT patch.

A few years ago, I faced an angry mob of volunteer first-aiders. They told me (in their own way) that mandatory EMT training would be a financial burden on them, and that they were too busy to devote 81 hours to a training program. By the time I finish this course, I will have logged more than 500 miles traveling to regular classes and make-ups. In addition to the hours spent in class, I will have devoted countless hours with my nose in a book. The expense and inconvenience are a tiny price to pay for this wonderful opportunity to expand my knowledge and renew some long-lost skills.

If I get through this course, I'll have a renewed sense of appreciation for those who exhibit their achievement on a shoulder patch, or who place an "REMTA" after their name. If their EMT course was as good (and tough) as mine, they have plenty to be proud of. But I'll probably be more intolerant than ever of those who treat emergency care as a social activity. Those who want the opportunity to care for patients must be willing to accept the burdens of preparation and continual training.

When people refer to you as an "expert," it's easy to believe them. The diverse nature of EMS calls for many kinds of experts. But in prehospital care, there's only one kind of expert that counts — the person who can provide quality patient care "on the street." I'm looking forward to becoming a real expert. To do so, I must view my EMT course as just the beginning of a continual process of education and training.

POSTSCRIPT: This column appeared in the May, 1982 issue of JEMS. *That June I received my EMT certificate (whew!).*

The Magic of 3 a.m.

A few months after I had returned to this business of responding to emergencies,* my pager lifted me out of a sound sleep. Fumbling for the bedside light, trying to get my feet into waiting turnout pants, I heard the dispatcher say something about an overturned tank truck. Images of fireballs brought forth a surge of adrenalin. As I jogged to the garage, the dispatcher repeated the alarm, including the time.

. . . *"Your time out is 0300 hours."*

There it was again. That magical hour that is part and parcel of every good "war story" in EMS and the fire service. Have you ever noticed that the toughest extrications, the drunkest drunks, the deepest snow, and the biggest fires always happen at three o'clock in the morning? According to the war stories, that is.

******In August, 1984, I returned to the fire service to serve as a Battalion Chief for the Carlsbad, California, Fire Department.***

"It's 3 a.m., you've had 15 calls that shift, and 'ol 'Cadillac Jennie' fakes another heart attack down at the Lafayette Hotel. . . ."

Was it really 3 a.m.? Or was that just a little enhancement to the story? Could it be that magic hour — 180 minutes after midnight — has universal meaning to emergency personnel? Is that when we get our best sleep if not disturbed?

"You're just gettin' into that good sleep and they ring you out on a 'man down'. . . it's three o'clock in the morning."

I began to notice this phenomena several years ago while lecturing on EMS and the law. When it came time for the questions and answers, there would be an inevitable war story or several.

"We had this case a few months ago. . . it was three in the morning. . . ."

After I began to notice how many of the stories were presented in the context of that awful hour, I would get distracted. I would find myself wondering whether the case in question really did happen at 3 a.m. If not, is it really fair to the clock to hang all those bad stories on that one lonely hour? Who started this campaign against 0300 hours anyway?

"I really need a transfer, chief. I just can't handle getting up and going on all these calls at three in the morning."

Well, anyway, I was heading toward this reported overturned tank truck, looking toward the horizon for the tell-tale glow, listening to the radio for a report on conditions. Finally, it came. . . .

"*. . . overturned* trash *truck, no fire, no injuries, cancel other units.*"

With a little enhancement, that could make a pretty good war story. . . .

. . . *"So the alarm came in while I was sound asleep — it was 3 a.m. — and the dispatcher's voice was quaking as she reported an overturned tank truck."*

Would the story be half as good if it had happened at 11:30 p.m. or 5 a.m.? I don't know, but I thought about it as I shut off the lights and siren. I decided to take a tour of my city before going back to bed. I wanted to see what really happens at the mystical morning hour of three.

A lot of people are up and functioning between midnight and sunrise — delivering papers, cleaning banks, sweeping parking lots, driving buses. I wonder if they tell stories about odd things that happen to them at 3 a.m. Probably not. More likely, night people tell war stories about things that happen at noon.

This whole episode brought me to a conclusion. It's time we stopped picking on one solitary hour to reinforce stories that probably aren't true in the first place. Three a.m. has been bad-rapped too long and it deserves a break.

"It was three in the morning and I couldn't sleep. I was overdue on my deadline for 'The Publisher's Page' and I didn't know what to write about. I looked at the clock and there it was!"

Now, if the neighbor's cats will just finish their noisy romance, I may be able to get some sleep before the sun comes up.

POSTSCRIPT: After this column appeared in JEMS, *Peter King of Fontana, Wisconsin, wrote to say that he was reminded of the following quotation from F. Scott Fitzgerald: "In the dark night of the soul, it is always 3 o'clock in the morning."*

2

Battling the Bureaucracy

Purple Defiance

Bobby Gene was out behind the corn crib, planting potatoes, when Carol Sue hollered from the house.

"Sheriff's on the phone," she shouted.

"What's he want?" her husband shouted back.

"He says some guy from the State's down at the squad buildin'."

Bobby Gene had a day off from his job at the mill and he was using the free time and good weather to get the family garden in shape. His wife continued to shout from the house. "Wants to see somebody in charge — right away,"

He wiped his sweaty forehead and started slogging toward the house. As he arrived at the back porch, Carol Sue handed him a glass of iced tea. After drinking half the contents in one swig, Bobby Gene spoke as he scraped mud from his boots.

"Sheriff say what's the hurry?"

"He just said some guy from State EMS's down at the

squad buildin'."

"They don't never come out here from the State Capital less'n there's trouble," the sturdy man muttered.

"Whatcha reckon it's all about?" his wife asked.

Bobby Gene didn't answer. He finished the tea in another swig, placed the glass on the porch rail, and walked toward his pickup truck. As he climbed into the truck he had some parting instructions for Carol Sue.

"Call Elmer — tell him to meet me down at the squad buildin'."

As he drove the mile-and-a-half from his small farm to the volunteer rescue squad building, Bobby Gene pondered the possible reasons for the visit by the State EMS agency. He'd been Rescue Chief for three years and everything was in order, as far as he knew. All the members were EMT-trained, continuing education records were current, ambulance vehicles were licensed, and the State had inspected everything just a few months earlier. The squad building loomed in the distance as Bobby Gene was struck by a thought.

Harley Barton is a good EMT and a valuable member of the rescue squad, by most accounts. But he's had this problem with drinking. A few weeks earlier, he'd gone to an extrication course at the State Capital. After hours, he'd gone with a group to a local gin mill. After too much drinking Harley had expressed his undying love for the barmaid and then proceeded to prove it to the girl's boyfriend. The battle — and the consequent encounter with police officers — had made the front page of the *Capital City Times* the next day.

As he pulled into the parking lot, Bobby Gene was planning his explanation. He would tell the State EMS people Harley was a good EMT — Harley realizes he had a problem with booze — he's never going to drink again

— he apologized to the barmaid and her boyfriend and paid a stiff fine for his behavior. If the State EMS folks would let Harley keep his EMT certificate, the whole squad would vouch for his good behavior in the future.

Parking his pickup in the lot next to the squad building, Bobby Gene spotted a Ford Fairmont with federal license plates. Two men dressed in business suits started to get out of the Ford as soon as they spotted Bobby Gene. They walked toward him.

"Howdy," Bobby Gene said, as the two men approached.

The larger of the two men spoke first, introduced himself as a representative of the State EMS office. He introduced the other man as a U.S. Attorney.

U.S. *Attorney*! Bobby Gene thought. Harley made some trouble but it wasn't a federal offense, was it?

"What can I do for you?" he asked.

The attorney answered, "We'd like to look at your ambulances."

Bobby Gene shrugged and started fishing keys from a pocket of his coveralls. As the two men followed him to the building, the Rescue Chief stopped, turned, and asked, "This got anything to do with Harley Barton?"

The two men nodded negatively. As he unlocked the roll-up door at the front of the squad building, Bobby Gene was confused. "If they ain't here about Harley . . . what the hell they wanna look at the ambulances for. . . ."

He moved along the series of roll-up doors, unlocking and lifting them as he progressed. As the doors slid up, the bright sun reflected off the glistening ambulances parked inside. Two Type III Fords and a Type II Chevy, purchased with community donations and the proceeds of raffles and cake sales. In keeping with the volunteer Squad's tradition, all three vehicles had been repainted with several coats of hand-rubbed purple lacquer.

The government lawyer frowned as he walked between the vehicles and peered at their rear windows. He pulled a small notebook from his pocket and started to write. Bobby Gene watched silently. As the lawyer moved from vehicle to vehicle, jotting notes in his book, Elmer Burns huffed into the building at a half-running pace.

"What's up, Bobby Gene, what is it?"

"Dunno, Elmer. This here's a U.S. lawyer an' he wanted to see the ambulances."

Elmer stepped toward the lawyer, who was intent on his notebook. "I'm Elmer Burns, County Commissioner and lawyer myself by trade. What's the problem?"

The government lawyer stopped writing in his notebook, shook Elmer's hand, and pointed to the rear of one of the ambulances.

"I'm here at the request of the regional office of the National Highway Traffic Safety Administration. I received a complaint about your ambulances. Under federal law, if an ambulance vehicle does not comply with federal standards and specifications. . . ."

Elmer Burn's jaw dropped in disbelief.

"Whaddayamean, *don't comply*? I can show you the paperwork. *All* of them ambulances meet your dadgum Gee Ess Aye, Yoo Ess Aye, Enn Aych Tee Ess Aye an' Kay Kay Kay riggamoroles. What more do you want?"

"I don't know anything about that," the government lawyer said officially. "All I know is that these vehicles are in violation of Section Three, Point One Six, Point Three of Federal Specification, Ambulance, dated Two January, Nineteen Seventy Four."

"Whatcha mean, in violation?" Elmer demanded angrily.

The government lawyer responded with cool authority.

"According to the Federal Specification, these vehicles must be painted standard gloss white with a orange band or stripe not less nor more than fourteen inches wide encircling the entire ambulance body configuration at the belt line as a condition for displaying the registered "Star of Life" symbol, you see," and he pointed to the "star."

Pudgy Elmer Burns, shirt-tail hanging out, hands on hips, tousled hair falling across his forehead, looked up at the government lawyer through squinting eyes. Defiance dripped from his words as he spoke after a long pause.

"The — hell — you — say."

Five Years Later

WASHINGTON, D.C. — The federal government's efforts to use trade-mark laws to regulate the color of ambulances received a sharp setback, according to a Supreme Court decision yesterday. A unanimous Court ruled in favor of the Dismal Seepage Volunteer Rescue Squad in its five-year battle with the U.S. Department of Transportation. In an opinion written by the Chief Justice, the Court ruled that use of trade-mark legislation and registration for such far-ranging regulatory purposes "stretches beyond rational explanation the Congress' intent in creating an important tool for the protection and regulation of commerce."

At issue was a symbol known as the "Star of Life," often affixed to ambulance vehicles. The symbol had been registered with the Commissioner of Patents and Trade Marks in 1977. In 1980, the Department of Transportation had issued a "get tough" memo urging its regional offices to take legal action against those who displayed the "Star of Life" on vehicles not conforming to the federal government's ambulance specifications, including color scheme.

The Court's opinion stated: "The Constitution gives Congress the power 'To regulate Commerce with foreign Nations, and among the several States, and with the Indian Tribes.' If living today, the framers of that Constitutional provision surely would lapse into cardiac arrest were they to witness the repugnant efforts of a federal agency to influence and control the color of motor vehicles through this imaginative but dangerous extension of power."

The Court's ruling was more than a symbolic victory for the small town of Dismal Seepage and for Elmer Burns, the self-styled "country lawyer" who pursued the case through the legal system for more than five years.

Burns held a press conference in a Washington hotel to announce his candidacy for President of the United States. Among his proposed domestic policies was a proposal to paint all ambulances purple and to equip those vehicles with a symbol called the "Square of Life."

POSTSCRIPT: This piece was written under the pseudonym, "Sinclair Germaine." Sinclair was born in the midst of an all-night work session during my first months as a magazine publisher. Nothing had prepared me for the pressures of creating an under-financed magazine and introducing it to a crowded field in the middle of a serious recession. Possibly as a defense against stress, my eccentric alter-ego emerged. His mission: Puncture pomposity, expose the ridiculous, and go public with some messages that were a little too hot for me to handle.

The preceding fictional account appeared in JEMS *in August, 1980. Since then the issue of ambulance colors seems to have gone the way of Sinclair Germaine (last seen riding his bicycle into a Bolivian sunset). As I travel around the U.S., the ingenuity and independence of EMS and fire service folks is apparent in the paint schemes on their ambulances. At last report, the federal government has never tried to enforce its ambulance color standard through legal action. The role model for Elmer Burns continues to pose as a politician in North Carolina.*

On Target

Most of us would like to see our nation's newspapers give more space and attention to the problems of emergency medical care. All too often, when the topic is covered, it's fragmentary or overlooks the real problems. But when a newspaper hits the target and hits it hard, it's worth some praise.

Recently, a daily newspaper in a major U.S. city published a series of editorials about that community's happenstance approach to caring for seriously injured people. We won't mention the newspaper or the city, because that would merely suggest that the city in question is worse off than most; it isn't.

The first editorial was called "Death in the Golden Hour." It started with a description of an accident — a man had fallen from a 200-foot cliff onto rock at the edge of a body of water. He had a significant head injury and wasn't breathing.

"The paramedics rappelled down the cliff to reach him.

On the hillside, they started IVs, pumped up shock trousers to keep his circulation going, resuscitated him and carried him down to the beach.

"A helicopter hovered over the injured man and hoisted him up to the aircraft. He was then flown to the most appropriate hospital where a specially trained trauma team treated his multiple injuries.

"The man has made a complete recovery. . . This is the kind of story paramedics like to tell, while waiting for an emergency call. They don't like to tell about the trauma victims who were taken to a hospital that didn't have the facilities to care for victims with multiple injuries. They don't like to tell about the young people who are paralyzed today because, when they were being treated for a chest wound in an understaffed emergency room, the doctor didn't have a diagnostic CAT scan to know they had also suffered spinal column injuries. They don't like to tell about the people who died on the table in a satellite hospital, when they could have survived in a major hospital set up for trauma a few minutes away.

"The paramedics don't like to tell the horror stories because they know they can happen again. Today. To somebody's grandmother who's been run over on a street. Or somebody's son who has hurtled out of control on a motorcycle. Because (name of city) does not have a trauma system that selects the trauma victim with multiple injuries from other emergency cases and directs him to the trauma unit that may save him. It doesn't have a system that designates hospitals with trauma units and says other hospitals shouldn't handle major trauma. It doesn't have a system that delivers all victims within the golden hour paramedics have to stabilize a trauma patient and get him to an appropriate surgeon before he dies or becomes a vegetable."

The editorial then criticized a "vague rule" in its home city that requires the victim to be taken to the closest hospital. "The rule makes sense for most medical emergencies. Heart attacks, strokes, breathing problems can usually be treated in emergency rooms of both small and large hospitals. The rule makes sense for minor trauma injuries, such as broken limbs.

"But it makes no sense for a victim of major trauma with multiple injuries to the head, body and limbs to be sent to a hospital that has no surgeon on duty, no CAT scanner, no heart pump, no team of doctors, nurses and technicians who are trained to work on several injuries at once.

"This usually doesn't happen. Usually, the hospital without trauma facilities will tell an ambulance with a major trauma victim to pass it by. But it can happen. And when it does, the people involved don't forget it. They don't like to talk about it, because they don't like to resuscitate people in order for them to die in the hospital."

We couldn't have said it better. Not only is it refreshing to see a newspaper identify a real problem and attack it, but we appreciate their stating it from the point of view of the people who must care for the victim in the street.

As you've read this, you've probably wondered what city the newspaper was referring to. Many readers, in different cities, will recognize the issues as their own. Perhaps it's time they educated *their* local media representatives.

An Open Letter to the President

Dear Mr. President: Like many others, I've been worrying about world peace and our military establishment. Sometimes I want to believe that massive defense spending will make our nation and the world a safer place. Other times, the efforts of nations to intimidate one another seems to me insane at best.

My skepticism peaks every time I have a close encounter with Pentagon thinking. The most recent episode of doubt occurred as I toured an ambulance assembly line. There I saw ambulances being built for the U.S. Army and Navy.

Ten years ago, the federal government published minimum design and performance standards for ambulance vehicles. They were made mandatory for all ambulances purchased with federal funds, and a majority of states also have adopted them.

Though there are limits imposed by the truck and van chassis of the three major auto manufacturers, the modern ambulance — built to federal specifications — is efficient, relatively economical, and effective as a patient care and transportation vehicle. Ambulance builders through the last decade continuously have fine-tuned it. The federal specification has become the standard for emergency medical transportation. Almost.

While three branches of your federal government (GSA, DOT and HHS) have insisted on compliance with the federal ambulance specification, another branch (Defense) has ignored it. The Army and Navy ambulances on the assembly line are a perfect example.

To meet the military specs, the ambulance builder was forced to use the least appropriate chassis available. Exterior colors are white with an orange stripe, but that's where the similarities end. For example, painted numbers and letters on the Navy vehicle are blue. The Army requires them to be black. The Navy specifies an orange cross insignia. The Army's cross is red. In the Navy ambulance, the radio control head and microphone are mounted overhead. In the Army ambulance it's mounted on the rear of the engine cover near the floor.

The Army requires a stationary, wall-mounted, electric suction unit. The Navy specifies a portable suction unit, strapped to an interior wall. The Army calls for an upright cabinet at the front bulkhead of the patient compartment. The Navy specifies a lateral squad bench at that position.

Both versions of the military ambulance have fluorescent overhead lights, which are extra cost items not considered necessary in the federal (GSA) specifications. Both are equipped with a tubular steel "cow catcher" arrangement forward of the front bumper. On that device — out where they will be in contact with everything — the Army and Navy demand that warning lights with plastic lenses be mounted. (We'd be interested in the replacement lens concession.) Another thing that's common to both ambulances is a flat steel plate affixed to the top of the exhaust pipes as they emerge from the left rear corner of the vehicle. The brass was concerned that spilled gas on hot pipes would be a fire hazard. But won't a steel plate mounted to an exhaust pipe get as hot as the pipe itself? And won't the flat plate serve as a nice step or foot rest? (We'd also be interested in the replacement exhaust pipe concession.)

But here's the worst part, Mr. President. The Army, the Navy *and* the GSA have sent high-level people to inspect the ambulances in production. They have traveled long distances at great expense to make sure the Department of Defense buys ambulance vehicles that are dissimilar, that don't meet the GSA's own specifications, that are built on the least suitable chassis, that have safety hazards resulting from poor military design and that cost more than a top-of-the-line civilian ambulance of similar type.

Back to the original point, I'm convinced that the Pentagon is brimming with people who don't have enough to do, people who continuously look for ways to justify their position (like designing ambulances to be overpriced, inefficient and hazardous).

Are ambulances an exception, Mr. President, or do your folks at the Pentagon play the same game with planes, tanks, missiles and rifles? If they find it necessary to justify their positions, can we believe that they don't sometimes hope for a little war?

POSTSCRIPT: This column appeared in the April, 1984 issue of JEMS. A copy was included in a package the General Services Administration sent to Congress to spur action in this area. We are told that military specifications for ambulances are much closer today to the GSA specifications (KKK-A-1822B), except for differences in interior layout. While that effort is commendable, I still worry when I read of $600 ashtrays and $60 screwdrivers for the military.

Maneuvering Around Heimlich

For longer than we like to remember, most Americans who've been paying attention have been entertained by the spectacular combat between Henry Heimlich, M.D., the Red Cross, the National Academy of Science, the American Heart Association, and... (it seems like there were others).

"Entertained?" Yes, as in "attending a bullfight." We don't have to recount the history. It's been adequately reported in the press. Besides, if you don't already know about the conflict, you probably stopped reading this article in the first paragraph.

A "bore" was once described as a person who continues to tell you about something long after you've lost interest. Let's face it. The "Heimlich controversy" has become boring.

What's that you say? It's a matter of life or death to 3,000 people every year? Well, we killed that many people on our streets and highways every 22.6 days last year. Try to talk ABC or CBS into a prime-time story about highway deaths, drinking and driving, passive restraints, or enforcement of the double nickel.

The "Heimlich controversy" has been visible and topical because it includes an emotional battle between people who are supposed to be *un*emotional . . . at least when it comes to their profession. Flat-out public controversies between medical scientists don't happen all that often. The last to rival Heimlich versus The Establishment was the Salk versus Sabin battle over whose polio vaccine was best. But in time, we get tired of all the fine points of debate advanced by one side and then the other.

Relief is in sight. It all happened in Dallas on September 19th and 20th.* A compromise of sorts was reached. The event was the 1979 National Conference on Standards for CPR and Emergency Cardiac Care, held at the Heart Association's National Center. But the compromise may have its origins in another earlier meeting.

It was the Disneyland Hotel in Anaheim, July 23, 1979. The ACT Foundation's committee of medical advisors was holding one of its once-in-a-while informal meetings. Chairing the session was Professor James V. Warren, M.D., godfather of Columbus' paramedics and a former president of the American Heart Association. Also in attendance was Leonard A. Cobb, M.D., grand mogul of the Seattle EMS System, and Stephen Carveth, M.D., long-time hard worker in the AHA's Emergency Cardiac Care Committee, chairman of Nebraska's giant CPR training campaign, and a cardiovascular surgeon in

---

**This article appeared in the Fall, 1979 issue of Paramedics International, (predecessor to* JEMS *) under the Sinclair Germaine pseudonym. In July, 1985 the National Conference on Standards and Guidelines for CPR and Emergency Cardiac Care again met. The results will be discussed in a postscript to this piece.*

Lincoln. The "Heimlich controversy" was on the agenda.

"It's simple," said Cobb, as heads turned in querulous amazement. "Why not just reverse the sequence?," he asked. Expanding on his suggestion in matter-of-fact tones, Dr. Cobb said, "If he's right (referring to Dr. Heimlich's contention that the manual thrust, otherwise known as the "Heimlich technique," is the *only* technique to be used), there will never be a need to do the back slaps."

The sequel was obvious. If the manual thrusts don't work in a given case, the rescuer could revert to back slaps. Since no party to the controversy had advanced any conclusive data to support their positions, who could argue with this minor amendment?

The Anaheim meeting ended with a sense that history had been made . . . right across the street from tomorrowland. One of the committee members was to advance the proposal to the right folks. But in the days that followed, hostility between the adversaries intensified, lawsuits were being threatened, and there was even some talk of a Congressional investigation (yawn).

Nobody got too excited when the reversed-sequence proposal went into limbo. After all, the Dallas meeting was coming up and Heimlich himself was among the invitees. Some saw this event as *the* opportunity to settle the issue, once and for all. Others anticipated the event in terms normally reserved for boxing matches.

On September 17th, word leaked that Heimlich wasn't going to attend the conference in Dallas. Trevor Hughes, M.D., formerly of the University of North Carolina and now a California anesthesiologist, heard that the Heimlich seat would be empty and asked for the opportunity to attend in his place. Hughes, a vocal supporter of Heimlich, expressed the view that the meeting would be a "sham" if nobody was there to represent Heimlich's point of view.

The conference opened with a general session. Among the presenters was Dr. Joe Redding (University of South Carolina) who reported on his analysis of 225 cases of foreign body airway obstruction collected by the American Heart Association. Redding was direct and to-the-point. Generally, he reported that there is insufficient evidence to recommend any single measure (technique) to the exclusion of others, or to strongly condemn any measure. No single maneuver, when used alone, was classed as successful in more than half the cases studied, according to Dr. Redding. Summarily, he concluded, "Both the American Heart Association and Heimlich rely on anecdotal data."

Immediately following Dr. Redding's presentation, Myron Weisfeldt, M.D., was invited to make a presentation on his research at Johns Hopkins University. Speaking at machine gun pace, Dr. Weisfeldt painted a picture of the future of cardiopulmonary resuscitation. With slides to illustrate his revolutionary findings of the cardiovascular mechanism, he repeatedly stated that the research was not conclusive. But few doubted that the Johns Hopkins results would be duplicated elsewhere before long and that such changes as simultaneous compression and ventilation might find their way into CPR training in a few years. Puritanically scientific to the end, Dr. Weisfeldt concluded with the warning that the CPR technique should not be changed based on his data, and that any changes should be first tested through longer and more numerous scientific tests.

Few could put the "Heimlich controversy" on the back burner as Mike Weisfeldt did at Dallas. Particularly to the non-physicians in the audience, his presentation was little short of mind-boggling. But after lunch (soup and sandwich), the conference was scheduled to break into panels, including one entitled "Obstructed Airway."

Eugene L. Nagel, M.D., was the designated Chairman of the panel. Doctors Cobb and Carveth were also at the conference but assigned to other panels. We don't know whether there was an earlier meeting or conversation between the three at or before the conference. It could be that great minds often do travel the same paths. Whatever the path, it was Dr. Nagel who raised the possibility of a reversed sequence compromise.

But first there were some skirmishes of opinion. Dr. Hughes offered and described data collected by Heimlich and Dr. Harry Gibbons, totalling 488 cases of foreign body airway obstruction. Dr. Redding reemphasized that there is no known "best way" to address foreign body airway obstruction at this time; he urged that no single approach be emphasized over others until better data is available.

C.P. Dail, representing the Red Cross, reiterated his organization's reliance on the National Academy of Science for guidance on this and other medical matters. Dr. Archer Gordon, a member of the National Academy of Science committee which advises the Red Cross, offered information on current studies tending to show that back blows dislodge foreign bodies in the airway. He took issue with Heimlich's frequent statement that "back blows are death blows."

At this point, Nagel made his move. Trying to place things in perspective, he observed that the infamous disagreement is a relatively minor matter when compared to 300,000 pre-hospital cardiac deaths per year. He suggested that the controversy has been detrimental to public education efforts. The publicity over this issue, he commented, tends to overshadow the fact that 10,000 to 15,000 lives per year are saved from pre-hospital cardiac deaths by basic and advanced life support systems.

The spirit of compromise was in the air. Nagel's suggestion concerning a reversal of the sequence prompted one physician to say, "I would propose and accept a compromise in a minute if it would stop Heimlich's attacks on the American Heart Association and the Red Cross." The comment brought Hughes to his feet. "We shouldn't make revisions based on whether Heimlich agrees," he said. "If it's better (a revised technique or sequence), it should be incorporated in the Standards."

The tide toward compromise weakened briefly as one doctor commented that it would cost his local Heart Association affiliate $15,000 to print and mail new instructions to its instructors. Nagel moderated the argument with a comment that a negotiated resolution of *this* controversy might well be cost effective in the long run.

The day ended all too soon and the various panel members repaired to the Twin Sixties Hotel for more meeting and conferring. During the evening session, the compromise gained momentum. According to the prevalent rumor, Hughes phoned Heimlich and found him agreeable to the idea.

The next morning was programmed for reports from the various panels and discussion of those reports (presumably for adoption and inclusion in the revised Standards which will be published in a forthcoming Supplement to *JAMA (Journal of the American Medical Association*). When the obstructed airway report was presented, there was the expected suggestion that no single maneuver or technique be recommended alone, that a combination of techniques seems more reasonable in view of the lack of data.

Dr. Hughes made a strong statement for the "Heimlich" maneuver as the technique of choice. Nagel again took charge. "I would like to see some data on reversal of the procedure," he said. He then recommended that selected AHA affiliates test the reversed sequence for 12 to 18 months and then report their results. The suggestion was reaffirmed by Dr. Alan Brandt, of Milford, Connecticut.

At this point, one of the conferees, apparently unaware of the history being made, rose to demand that "we stop calling this the 'Heimlich' maneuver. We don't apply the names of Safar, Jude, Knickerbocker and Keuwenhoven to the techniques they devised," he said. The chairman skillfully got the meeting back on track.

Dr. Steve Carveth then rose to comment. He called for "open minds." He strongly urged the assembled medical leadership to create an appropriate atmosphere for a research organization to work with the Heart Association and Red Cross in studying either the back blow/manual thrust sequence *or* the manual thrust/back blow sequence. (He limited his suggestion to apply to only conscious upright victims.) Carveth's suggestion was supported by Nagel and by New Jersey cardiologist Klaus Schultz.

Red Cross representatives were quick to dissent. "If we make this an either/or proposition — let the public make up its own mind — it's going to confuse the public further," said one. Another Red Cross rep raised the issues of cost and credibility. "We have millions of dollars invested in text materials. We can't throw these materials away every time there is a change; so, we send out supplements. When people end up with more supplement materials than text materials, the credibility of the organization becomes questionable." Finalizing, he said, "We need a standard we can count on, modified every few years to reflect the state-of-the-art, and supported by scientific data."

Dr. Eugene Nagel had the last word: "We don't have enough data to reverse our position, but we also don't have enough data to resist reversal of the sequence — with training organizations studying the alternative in a controlled study." But possibly one of the more important statements was made by Joel Grottenthaler, Executive Director of Pennyslvania's Emergency Health Services Federation. He told the body, "People in the field aren't necessarily going to follow your mandate."

Although tainted by the absence of reliable data, there is a strong indication that trainers and trainees had made their decisions as to technique of choice long before the Dallas conference. There is additional evidence that others were on the fence, just waiting for somebody's data to prevail or for a compromise to surface. Most of those interviewed (in a nonscientific survey of an insignificant statistical sample of interviewees) reported that they knew what they would do when confronted by a person choking, but they refused to be quoted.

As history records the probable end of the "Heimlich controversy," it'll be interesting to read the footnote about Trevor Hughes. He was the only one of 100 attendees to openly represent Heimlich's point of view. The response to his attendance and participation could not be described as warm and friendly. It's doubtful that his persistent advocacy was all that persuasive. But without him, the meeting would have lacked any degree of credibility. No conference which presumes to rule on a hotly debated issue can succeed if only one side of the issue is presented.

Inordinate delay in publishing the new Standards is certain to see Dr. Heimlich commenting publicly on how he reads the compromise. If his version deviates in any way from the official (but unpublished) version, we might expect still another round of acrimony.

Before agreeing to print this article, the publisher submitted my draft to a number of "real people" (folks who rescue other folks as a profession, avocation, or voluntary service). The results of that survey were interesting. Many were not even aware of the controversy. Those who were aware of the controversy had already made their own decisions as to what they would do. None had any prior understanding of the process by which these matters are decided. Very few knew anything about the power structure of medical politics.

True scientists would scoff at such anecdotal data. But can they really afford to? Isn't it conceivable that this "controversy" has been little more than a few people fighting with a few people, presuming to be in the spotlight, while the "real people" went about their business oblivious to the medical politics? After the research, interviewing and writing that went into this article, I'm inclined to side with the "real people." Unless Heimlich and his adversaries can establish credibility with the rescuers of our country, and unless they can devise a method for communicating quickly and regularly with those rescuers on rescuer's terms, their respective efforts to serve as standard-setters will be so much unimportant hot air.

POSTSCRIPT: When the official standards were finally published in JAMA in August, 1980, the confusing "dual approach" was adopted, with the standard being to alternate back blows with abdominal thrusts (back blows first). The controversy did not die, and five more years of debate followed (although I'm sure the "real people" knew what to do.)

In July, 1985 the National Conference on Standards and Guidelines for CPR and Emergency Cardiac Care again met, and foreign body airway obstruction was again a topic. JEMS *Contributing Editor Mary Newman was there and reported that experts called for across-the-board endorsement of the Heimlich Maneuver. She wrote in the September, 1985 issue of* JEMS*: "While no further scientific studies were cited in support of the abdominal thrust, it is the feeling of the panel (of experts) that it would be unreasonable to continue to ignore the accumulation of six years of additional field experience* *demonstrating the successful use of this technique . . . conference leaders also indicated that the excessive attention that has been devoted to the Heimlich controversy may be counter-productive to the general aims of emergency cardiac care. . . . With these interests in mind, it was the majority recommendation of the panel to endorse the abdominal thrust as the exclusive treatment for all victims of foreign airway obstruction. The panel was unaware of any evidence to support the widely held assumption that the abdominal thrust cannot be used safely and effectively, even in cases of pregnancy and obesity." The panel included Dr. Roger White, MD, chairman, James Atkins, MD, Richard L. Day, MD, Joseph Greshler, MD, Henry Heimlich, MD, and Trevor Hughes, MD.*

When the revised guidelines were published in the June 6, 1986 issue of the Journal of the American Medical Association, those recommendations became official (except for infants, where back blows and chest thrusts are recommended). Has the Heimlich Controversy finally died as a footnote to the power, and the drain, of medical politics?

EMS Graffiti

"American Graffiti" notwithstanding, I remember the 1950s as an awful time to pass through puberty. I was too skinny for athletics, my car was forever broken, and I hated the tribal rituals of teen-age boys who hadn't yet distinguished their glands from their brains. The rituals reached a peak as we approached the homecoming football game against our cross-town rival high school.

On Monday before the Friday night game, we began to convince ourselves that the kids who attended Alhambra High School somehow were different from us. The mere mention of blue and gold (Alhambra's school colors) would generate subtle sensations of dislike. By Tuesday, the intolerance was less subtle; crudely drawn caricatures of A.H.S. football players would begin to appear on bulletin boards. On Wednesday, the art class would decorate the hallways with banners painted with provocative slogans ("Kill Alhambra").

Thursday usually presented us with tribal frenzy. One

or more of our gridiron stars would "deck" an unsuspecting student (or teacher) for failure to show sufficient deference to our football team (on whose shoulders rested the entire weight of our school's reputation.) But Friday was the ritual climax. For some strange reason, the school would schedule a "pep rally" on Friday morning. The result never varied. Those with the most severe cases of glandular confusion would pile into a fleet of '41 Fords and head for the campus of Alhambra High School to wage war on the opposing tribe. The football game always seemed anticlimatic.

As students, our mission was to prepare ourselves for carrying the world through another generation. But the mission got confused somehow as the vital juices of adulthood coursed through the bodies and brains of youth. At the last class reunion, it was interesting to note how many of those tribal warriors had managed to put things in proper perspective as they matured. Some of them even married graduates of Alhambra High School.

These recollections surfaced recently in the aftermath of a campaign to promote one form of prehospital EMS, discredit another form, and ignore all the others. Instinctively, the tribes surfaced. Intolerance for those who were somehow different marked the EMS gossip, the meetings and conferences, and the long-distance phone calls.

One outspoken individual buttonholed me at a meeting. He started the conversation with a question, but he really wasn't looking for an answer. Before I could utter a half dozen words, he unleashed a stream of vitriol about people who provide EMS through a profile different than his own. Before he was finished, he revealed his true concern. It had nothing to do with patient care.

A few days later, I heard from someone who believed

in a different method for delivering prehospital EMS. He had some unkind things to say about the folks who do not do it his way. But the capper was an anonymous note I received from somebody in Kansas. We were accused of "catering" to one type of delivery system while ignoring the others.

All they needed was a pep rally and a '41 Ford. They were ready to invade one another's campus. Their mutual mission — caring for sick and injured people to the best of their abilities — somehow got confused as the vital juices of youth coursed through the bodies and brains of adults. It was Friday afternoon all over again.

In recent years, we've preached long and loud for prehospital "street people" (first responders, EMTs, paramedics) to seek out and accept medical leadership. We've felt that an infusion of professional maturity and clarity of mission would result from a close working relationship between the street people and their physician mentors. We felt the doctors could set an example. More recently, we note that the current wave of tribal warfare among prehospital providers was preceded by public squabbling and carping among some of the medical specialty groups. Some example!

C'mon fellas, there's enough room — and action — for everybody. Let's tear down the pep-rally banners. There is absolutely no way that sharp rivalry among private ambulance people, fire department types, and "Third Service" devotees can produce any tangible benefits for patients.

Lemons into Creampuffs

A few years ago, the Chrysler Corporation found itself face-to-face with excess overhead and a national recession. The solution: get rid of a bunch of engineers. Chrysler saved some salary money, but it set the stage for an economic crisis. Five years later, Chrysler was building poorly designed, poorly built, pigs.

When some Arabs in the Middle East shut off the oil in '74, my boss (a political hopeful) in North Carolina ordered that our full-size State cars (16.5 mpg) be traded in for a fleet of Valiants (12 mpg). He lost the next election. There is some justice.

Chrysler went on underestimating the public. They subjected us to the Aspen and Volare. In 1978, I was part of a riot at the Avis counter at San Francisco International Airport. More than a dozen of us had been subjected to the bad habits of Chrysler's compact pigs. Mine died with every right turn. Avis cancelled its contract with Chrysler and Chrysler hired the ultimate paramedic — Lee Iacoca

— to save it from the corporate equivalent of ventricular fibrillation.

As we all know, the government stepped in to save Chrysler. Paramedic Iacoca has proved to be a terrific patients' advocate.

We have an analogous situation in EMS. Eight years ago,* the Congress dangled before us the promise of a major national initiative to improve EMS throughout the U.S. They passed a law mandating the Department of Health, Education and Welfare (DHEW) to build regional systems from coast-to-coast. DHEW decided to save some salary money and never hired any engineers.

They gave us a helluva ad campaign. "Designate a trauma center and get a check!" But the explanations for medical control (X, Y and Y prime) resembled a Dodge Diplomat (an Aspen by any other name. . .). DHEW borrowed from the success of Chrysler's "push button drive" when it decided to design a radio communications technology. For mileage figures, Chrysler got some meaningless numbers from the EPA. With a few notable exceptions, DHEW blew several million on EMS research that only proved the grant-writing aptitude of academic "good ol' boys."

Despite their many faults, Chrysler's four-wheeled pigs moved millions of people billions of miles between breakdowns, stall-outs, rattles, squeaks and sagging springs. At the same time, the federal government's EMS initiative has saved untold numbers of lives. But it could have done so much more without all the design defects.

Chrysler got bailed out by the government. But the government wasn't so generous with its own EMS program. It was traded in for an F-16 fighter and

---

**This article appeared in the October, 1981 issue of* JEMS.

an M-1 tank (built by Chrysler).

So it's up to us to turn lemons into creampuffs. I once owned a Renault Dauphine with a turbo-charged Corvair engine and transaxle. Anything is possible. We can take the remnants of DHEW's EMS campaign and build a precision life-saving machine. But not if we continue to argue over hood ornaments and hubcaps.

The main purpose of an automobile is to move the driver and passengers from point A to point B reliably, safely and with minimal effort. The main purpose of an EMS system is to provide for *all* of the emergency patient's needs reliably — whether or not he is capable of thinking or acting for himself.

It's a matter of engineering and competent driving. If the Congress leaves us with a faulty vehicle, we'll just have to rebuild it till it performs properly. As we go about rebuilding, we should remember that no amount of chrome, velour, vinyl, advertising, or rebate checks can substitute for reliable performance.

Meanwhile, it would be unfair to not recognize the hard work and sincere dedication of many people who were employed in the campaign to improve EMS since 1973. We had the pleasure of meeting most of them and we found only a few who were along just for the ride. From the leadership in Washington to the regional coordinators throughout the nation, there was a spirit of commitment seldom found in government programs. Even though some troubling errors occurred in the process, it was refreshing to be witness to and a part of the federal EMS initiative.

The Power of the Podium

About a year ago, a famous trauma surgeon visited the surgical society in a medium-sized city in one of our more populous states. He was the featured speaker at the monthly meeting of the group. Attendance at the meeting was better than usual; the speaker was a celebrity of sorts and the subject of his speech (trauma) was topical.

"Get your paramedics under control," said the doctor, in essence, "or, better yet, get rid of them." Since paramedics had been the brainchildren of cardiologists, few surgeons have ever really cottoned to the idea of prehospital advanced life support. "Don't let them fool around with the patient in the field," the surgeon told his rapt audience. "The only place you'll save the trauma patient is on the operating table, and all you need to get them there is rapid transportation."

We've paraphrased the famous surgeon, but we've accurately portrayed the message as it was received by the local surgeons. A few months later, we visited the city in question. The local surgeons had picked up the gauntlet and they were urging a dismantling of the local paramedic service. Of course, the citizens of the community generally were unaware of the growing controversy. In the meantime, paramedics and emergency physicians were scrambling to preserve the system they had built during the prior decade.

Can it be true, as the visiting surgeon suggested, that overzealous paramedics, superenthused by their minimal training, are actually killing patients by "fooling around" with them in the field when they really need to be on the operating table? Is it reasonable to suggest that paramedic systems be scrapped in favor of the old scoop-and-run method of ambulance transport?

We spent some time looking at the records of the community's prehospital emergencies before passing judgment on the famous surgeon's provocative argument. In the three years prior to his visit, 1.3 percent of the total patients seen by paramedics fit into the category of major trauma (based on CRAMS Scores, Champion Trauma Scores, and Glasgow Coma Scales).

Then we looked at the performance of paramedics in those confirmed cases of traumatic injury. We researched the times spent at the scene and in transit to the hospital (the total time from arrival at scene until delivery of the patient to the hospital). The range of times was from three minutes to 34 minutes, and that included time spent on extrication. The average time was less than 18 minutes.

Right away, it was obvious that an out-of-town surgeon, bent on some kind of misinformed mission of revolution, had placed in jeopardy a system that had been in place for nearly 10 years. The public was greatly pleased with the system, and they repeatedly approved a tax levy to support it. But, without benefit of accurate information, a dynamic speaker with a powerful reputation had succeeded in placing the system on the defensive though the system had nothing to be ashamed of.

A podium can be a powerful place. Those who have the occasional privilege of podia have an obligation to get the facts straight, and in balance. When their opinions are submitted for publication, medical scientists (including surgeons) are scrupulous to base their opinions on statistical data and documented patient outcomes. No less a standard should apply to speaking presentations, particularly when they are aimed at revolutionary change (or regression) in prehospital care.

A major segment of the medical community never has been happy with prehospital advanced life support delivered by *non*-physicians. In days of physician shortages and ever-upward personal income, paramedics were tolerated. But this is the age of cost containment and the next decade is expected to introduce us to physician surpluses (up to 70,000 surplus physicians by 1990). Paramedics should brace for more misinformed missions of revolution.

In the example mentioned above, the paramedics and their supervisors had created an easy solution. The paramedics had diligently compiled good reports on the cases they handled. Their supervisor regularly had assembled that report information into summaries of data. They know what their system is doing and how it is performing.

Improved methods of caring for and transporting the life-threatened trauma patient should be a mutual goal for all of us. Working together in an atmosphere of education, cooperation and change based on solid evidence, we *can* make a difference. There is no place in that constructive environment for the loose-lipped grandstander who buzzes from town to town with glib but erroneous after-dinner speeches.

It's reasonable to presume that there are prehospital providers (both basic and advanced life support) who spend too much time "fooling around" with trauma patients in the field. The answer to that problem is greater physician involvement with those services, and improved education guidance.

How would you fare if the famous surgeon came to your town and encouraged a dismantling of your system? Would you have the solid information to prove him wrong? Building the necessary information base starts with each run report.

In any event, a battle of words and ideas countered by a presentation of argumentative data leaves the patient as the pawn. In all areas of emergency care, but especially in trauma care, teamwork is essential. However entertaining, the admonition to "get rid of" one segment or another of EMS (without unimpeachable data to support the admonition) can only detract from the needs of the only legitimate beneficiary of the system.

POSTSCRIPT: Possibly bored with the topic, the superstars of trauma surgery seem to have gone on to other controversies since 1984. Meantime, personal computers are popping up in EMS agencies from coast to coast — and EMTs are filling them with response time data and other information. In my view, the controversy was placed in proper perspective by paramedic Richard Feldman when he published the results of a well-designed study in the August '86 issue of JEMS *("Prehospital Intravenous Line Placement: A Time Study").*

Initially Yours

"I'm looking for a more challenging job," my friend said, "but I can't even get an interview without some graduate degree." I knew the feeling. Several years ago, before resigning myself to the poverty and insecurity of a writer, I had offered my talents to the world of EMS administration. A new federal program had been announced, millions of dollars were being offered to develop regional EMS systems, and I *knew* that I had the talent and energy to pilot such a project. I didn't even care where it was.

Night after night, I labored at my ancient Underwood, creating the most impressive resume yet devised. Strategically, I sprinkled hints of my virtues throughout this document of supreme self-service. Words like "intelligent," "articulate" and "competent" were placed

---

NOTE: This appeared originally under the byline of Sinclair Germaine, my eccentric alter ego.

with great care as I struggled to lead the prospective reader to the conclusion that I was the only person for the job (whatever it was).

Finally, the masterpiece was finished. Surely, I thought, the reader's eye would flow smoothly through the section on "Personal Data" to the section on "Experience" without even noticing that there was no section on "Education." After all, I had labeled this thing a "Curriculum Vitae." Any potential employer would surely recognize that as a sign of time well spent in academia (resumes are for commoners).

After selling my stereo to raise some quick cash, I took my "C.V." to Angie's Secretarial Service for retyping on an IBM Selectric and duplication on some heavy, buff-colored paper. With the leftover funds, I bought a roll of postage stamps and started to dispatch my irresistible offer of servitude to every known potential employer of EMS administrator/organizers in America.

Nothing happened. Days passed with no response. The Feds announced their grants and many of them went to organizations I had covered with my wonderful document. Still no response. I started calling them on the phone (later, I had to sell my Raleigh 10-speed to pay the phone bill). "We received your Curriculum Vitae and we'll call you if we have an opening that fits your background and education," they said. They never called.

The people hired to fill those jobs all had a list of initials after their name. I didn't. Some of them did their jobs well. Lots of them failed miserably. If given the chance, I would have been the best of the bunch. I had the brains, the street savvy, the instinct for getting people to cooperate and work together, the ability to read fast and write well, and I would have worked 20 hours a day to make my EMS project a success. But I didn't get the chance. I didn't have those initials after my name.

A friend told me I should have faked it, that nobody really checks your academic credentials if you act like you've been to graduate school. It never occured to me (honesty is another of my virtues). Besides, I'm not sure how you're supposed to act if you've been to graduate school.

There I was, without music or transportation, deeply depressed by the reality that I would never have the chance to make my mark in the world of EMS. Then I got a freelance writing assignment to cover the American Hospital Association's Advanced Institute on Hospital Personnel Administration and Labor Relations in Houston. It was there, in Houston, that I met one of my alltime heroes: H. Dudley Dewhirst (he has some initials after his name but they're not really important).

"Curb credentialism!" Dewhirst challenged his attentive audience. He then defined "credentialism" as "excessive reliance on degrees, licenses, certification and diplomas in the making of organizational decisions." I started to applaud but stopped mid-clap as dirty looks darted my way.

"Credentialism is pervasive in almost all fields today," Mr. Dewhirst reported. "However, while it is creeping into most institutions, it seems to be galloping into the health care field." He then went on to state that this fetish for credentials is a major cause of many of the problems facing hospitals.

For example, he suggested that credentialism thwarts motivation by blocking upward mobility. I could identify with that. "By encouraging a new medical occupation for each new technological advance, credentialism results in overspecialization, and jobs become increasingly fragmented," he reported. "Workers want to do the whole job, not just a small, insignificant piece."

Everybody who's anybody in EMS knows that coordination of people and services and organizations is a key to consistent quality in emergency medical care. In Houston, H. Dudley Dewhirst reported that credentialism hinders coordination. For example, the tendency to create new occupations and positions with each new expansion in technology (rather than expand the roles and responsibilities of existing occupations and positions) simply produces an unworkable chain of command and communication. The victims: coordination of services and quality patient care.

Mr. Dewhirst added to his indictment of credentialism by asserting that it creates bureaucracy. He pointed to the increased supervisory expectations of those who have initials after their names. It makes sense. Once you get those initials, you feel like you should be supervising more people. If you haven't got enough people to supervise, you create a new level of bureaucracy. In the health care field, this has resulted in patient care being delivered increasingly by less skilled personnel.

"Credentialism creates conflict," he continued. Referring to the training one receives while pursuing the credentials, Dewhirst said, "Along with the theory and the practice, a set of values is learned. These values usually include the belief that one's profession is the most important, that one's training is better than that of other types of professionals and that, therefore, members of one's profession should play a greater role and have more responsibility." Continuing, he pointed out that when normal disagreements are fueled by each professional's belief that he has a better credential, the result often is "open warfare."

After detailing how credentialism adds unnecessarily to

the cost of health care, H. Dudley Dewhirst leveled a statement that still rings in my ears. "There is a real need to protect the public from opportunists who would pretend that they are competent when they are not." Instinctively, I thought of some credentialed but incompetent people who were hired while promising performers (like me) couldn't even get an interview.

Adding some balance to his presentation, the speaker urged that the problem is not that credentials requirements exist but that reliance on credentials is excessive. "The philosophy seems to be that, if some credentials requirements are good, more must be better."

That was more than five years ago. Flying back from Houston, I was convinced that H. Dudley Dewhirst's message would sweep the nation and that people and their talents would soon be seen as more important than initials after their names. When an edited version of Dewhirst's paper was published in *Hospitals* magazine (July 1, 1975, Volume 49), I was sure it would revolutionize hiring and promotional practices in the health care field.

It didn't happen. In fact, it seems like everyone has started to hang initials on their names. EMTs are doing it (it seems that an REMT-P is better than a REMT-A which is better than a simple EMT-A). Nurses are doing it (you haven't lived till you meet an RN, BSN, MSN, MICN). But I didn't realize we'd lost the battle until an EMS administrator/consultant handed me his card recently. He had no less than 21 initials after his name!

Meanwhile, having seen the handwriting on the wall, I married a girl who had a car, a stereo, and a good job. I went back to school and got my graduate degree. But it gives me only two initials after my name. How can I possibly compete against people with five, ten or even 21 initials?

But wait! There may be hope for the future. Several months ago, when I applied to *JEMS* for a columnist's position, I knew I was up against some tough competition. One of the applicants seemed to have the job in the bag. He had lots of initials after his name and he was an associate professor of journalism. Later, after I had got the job and the other fellow hadn't, I asked the publisher why. "Because he misspelled 'Curriculum Vitae.' "

Yes, ladies and gentlemen, there is still a place for competence. Speaking of competence, my friend who was looking for a more challenging job in EMS is still looking. If you might be interested in hiring an intelligent, articulate, sober nonsmoker, a competent, no nonsense innovator and leader to pioneer your new or proposed EMS system, drop me a line.

3

Ethics, Honor and Training

The Real Challenge

If you're involved in emergency medical care, you're affected by the subject of training. Other than contact with patients, no other subject affects everybody in EMS so universally.

As we compose each issue of *JEMS*, selecting from our files the outstanding articles on training, we have hoped to make some positive impact on both trainers and trainees. Still, there lurks in the background some widespread attitude problems that bother us — making us wonder whether anything we publish will make a dent in the problem.

The problem is indifference. It's most apparent in those who simply feel they already know all they want to know. It shows up in people who resist continuing education and recertification, claiming to one and all that proving one's competence to care for human life is an imposition. It seems to reach epidemic proportions when we realize that less than 10 percent of all EMTs and paramedics ever attend an optional educational conference, belong to a professional organization, or subscribe to an EMS-related journal.

Recently, our nation's educational system began to acknowledge that a generation of students is severely deficient in reading, math and other basic skills. Only after the problem became scandalous were practical solutions proposed and implemented. That seems to be an unfortunate characteristic of political life in North America. Problems must reach crisis proportions before practical solutions are taken seriously.

Are we sliding toward a similar crisis in EMS? Are we really satisfied with the skills and knowledge that new EMTs and paramedics take to the field after training? Are those new EMTs and paramedics as *dis*satisfied with their knowledge and skills as they should be? Do they view their license or certificate as evidence that they are as good at patient care as they need to be? Or, do they view it as a starting point, an invitation to enhance and build on the initial knowledge and skills so that they might eventually be as good as they can possibly be?

A few years ago, a study in a midwestern state evaluated the skills of several hundred EMTs. It was an indepth evaluation, including written exams, oral interviews and field evaluations. The conclusion was shocking: one in seven was so poorly trained that he represented a greater hazard to the patients than if he hadn't been present. The defective performances and results were not tilted toward any group, paid or volunteer EMTs. But there was a distinct relationship to the original training of each of those tested.

Exceptional EMT and paramedic instructors make the critical difference. The exceptional instructor recognizes (if only by instinct) that attitudes are just as important as exam scores. The exceptional instructor never forgets that the only valid purpose of training in EMS is to better serve sick and injured people who cannot care for themselves. The exceptional instructor leaves an indelible mark on his trainees — an example of professionalism that both career and volunteer trainees will mold their own attitudes around.

Our national educational system went awry when educators became so involved with the process of education that they overlooked the end product — basic skills for surviving and being productive in our society. The editors of *JEMS* have attended and reviewed many EMS training programs throughout the U.S. in recent years, and we feel that with the exception of a handful of quality training centers, the EMS education "system" (such as it is) also is going awry.

While hundreds of thousands graduated from EMS training programs with marginal skills and indifferent attitudes, the people and organizations who purport to be leaders in EMS education concentrate on the process of EMS training rather than the end product. More often than not, national standards mean nothing more than a level we prefer not to sink below.

The time has come for a renewal of the real spirit of EMS training. The key to that renewal is the individual instructor. No legislation, no state or federal bureaucracy or program can make the difference. National standards and programs of accreditation will go unnoticed by those who need the inspirational example of an exceptional instructor.

EMT and paramedic students must be motivated to recognize that the ultimate reward of their craft may be the comfort they can offer to an injured child or an elderly stroke victim. They must be inspired to exercise their intellectual curiosity — the driving compulsion to constantly improve and to learn as much as they possibly can about emergency care. They must be dissuaded from thinking of EMS as a prop for their social needs.

A few years ago, some of our nation's basic industries lost their intellectual curiosity in an atmosphere of self-satisfied indifference. Today's diminished auto and steel industries present us with an important lesson. We cannot afford to be deceived by the numbers of EMTs and paramedics. We cannot assume that the numbers translate to the necessary knowledge and skills — or attitudes.

EMS training in the U.S. has become somewhat of an industry. Thousands of people feed on the process of churning out new EMTs and paramedics. Getting trainees through a testing and certification process is no great achievement if they have no real appreciation for the human dimensions of providing emergency care and transportation in the real world. Receiving an EMT card or certificate is an empty achievement unless the recipient is inspired to continually seek out and learn as much as possible about this most noble of public pursuits.

Spare The Agony

About 18 months ago, I got a chance to return to the workaday world of emergency service providers. It had been more than 10 years since I'd worn a uniform, commanded an emergency, supervised a drill, or answered to a title. Much of it, I have found, is like riding a bicycle — you never really forget how.

On the other hand, lots of change occurred while I was out of uniform. The public we serve has some different notions about such matters as quality of life, and "the right to die with dignity." Earlier, the public applauded and supported our crusade to save every life in jeopardy, no matter the cost, regardless of the patient's opinion. It was their duty to survive and it was our duty to save them.

It's not so clear anymore, and two events during the last year have helped me to see the problem in complex extremes. It all started when Mrs. M called me to complain

---

NOTE: This appeared in the February, 1986 issue of JEMS.

that my paramedics hadn't done enough to save her husband's life. A day later, Mrs. G walked into my office and dropped a pile of hospital bills on my desk. My paramedics, she explained, should not have performed their medical heroics on her ailing husband; he wanted to die in peace, without incurring big medical bills.

Mrs. M had been married to her husband for 56 years. They had both been college professors. After raising their family, they traveled extensively and thoroughly enjoyed their life together. One night in his 77th year, Mr. M rose from bed to go to the bathroom. Later, his wife found him prone in the hallway. She dialed 9-1-1.

Mrs. G was about 20 years younger than her husband. They had married late in life and had no children. Once he reached 80 years of age, his health deteriorated. When he was lucid, he would tell his wife that he welcomed death and wanted to go peacefully. One day last year, she went shopping and asked a neighbor to check in on Mr. G. When the neighbor checked, the old man was slumped over in his wheelchair. She dialed 9-1-1.

First responders arrived at Mrs. M's house before the paramedics. They found the patient in a state of rigor mortis and concluded that no resuscitative effort should be made. When Mrs. M noticed that the rescuers were not administering to her husband, she said, "Aren't you going to do something?" One of the rescuers turned to her and said, "He's dead."

According to her doctor, Mrs. M went through all the classic stages of grief in the following eight months. She denied that her husband was dead. Later, she was absorbed by guilt. Finally, she became angry and that's when I heard from her. We've since become friends and she's getting on with her life.

When Mrs. G returned from the store, my paramedics

were just leaving with her husband. They had restored a functional rhythm at the scene and they were sure they would log another "save." As it turned out, Mr. G lived only a few more hours.

Mrs. G has little use for me or my paramedics. I've written to her doctor, trying to explain why things happened as they did. I tried to explain how he could help his elderly patients by giving them some information on how to control their destiny — to "die with dignity." He never bothered to answer.

In the early days of this business, we kept box scores for paramedic "saves." We would hand out awards to the paramedic teams who achieved the highest numbers. It was sort of like a sport. We were saving lives at any cost and it was okay.

There's an historic parallel for the situation we now find ourselves in. About 30 years ago, the people and the courts began to tell police officials it wasn't enough to simply enforce the law; it had to be done within the framework of people's rights. A lot of cops had trouble with that, and some still do.

Before we become the convenient targets of criticism for depriving people of the right to die with dignity, we need to actively pursue some logical solutions. This is a problem of patient and family education. Elderly and terminal patients and their families need to know what happens when they dial for emergency services. They need to know when to make the call and when not to.

At present, in most of our communities, physicians, nurses, social workers, clergymen and "discharge planners" are not adequately confronting the fact that not everyone wants his life saved. Mr. and Mrs. G were victims of this negligence and so were my paramedics.

Now that the bad part is over for Mrs. M, she can accept

the fact that her husband was not salvageable, but she'll never forget those cold and abrupt words, "He's dead." Just a slight softening of tone or inflection, just a moment of eye contact, just a tiny hint of personal concern, might have spared her months of agony.

This nice lady reminded me once again that every death in the family has more than one victim, and that sensitivity (unlike riding a bicycle) can be forgotten if not practiced.

A Performing Art

The young nurse was on her first tour of duty as a skill evaluator for a paramedic unit. She was bright and attractive, and the paramedics were doing their best to impress her with wit and stories about offbeat patients. About two hours into the shift, they received an alarm — a multiple-vehicle accident on the interstate.

The scene looked terrible, with several damaged cars strewn about and traffic backed up for a mile or two. The paramedics and the nurse quickly located and checked all the drivers and passengers. Surprisingly, there were no injuries. Meantime, the district fire chief was inching his way through the traffic to the scene.

As the chief arrived at the scene, one of the paramedics said something very funny, within earshot of the nurse. She laughed. The chief saw her laughing amid the *apparent* carnage, and the next several minutes were very unpleasant.

In his diatribe, the chief made a point we all need to

think about from time to time. To us, wrecked cars, burning buildings and dying people are the normal working environment. To onlookers, those scenes are filled with dread and fear, solemn occasions where smiles, jokes and gallows humor are terribly inappropriate.

In another scene, a fire company rolled to a reported heart attack. One of the firefighters was working an overtime shift; normally he was assigned to a unit across town. A paramedic ambulance arrived a few minutes after the fire company. One of the paramedics was an old friend of the overtime firefighter. The patient, Mrs. Murphy, had been dead for several hours.

As they picked up equipment and carried it out to the rigs, the paramedic and the overtime firefighter renewed their friendship, recalling old times and swapping stories about good times past. Witnessing this from the sidewalk were Mrs. Murphy's neighbors of more than 40 years. What could possibly be so funny about the death of a neighbor and friend, they thought.

Recently, we've seen some press photos of EMTs and paramedics in action. Few of them were fit to print in *JEMS*. Like the picture of a funeral home ambulance crew in Henderson, Texas, moving an injured pedestrian onto a gurney without a backboard or cervical collar (the man had suffered a concussion, dislocated shoulder, broken arm, broken leg and broken kneecap). Or the picture in the *New York Times* of CPR being performed with horribly incorrect hand position.

Which brings us to the point of all this. If we could record our prehospital performances on film or videotape, how many of us would be proud of the picture? If we could see ourselves in public, in our official roles, as the public sees us, would we want to share those same images with our families, friends, bosses or fellow workers?

Many ingenious methods have been devised to monitor skills and assure the quality of EMT and paramedic performances. Based on the photos we've seen of some of those performances in places all over North America, some new methods are needed. To be sure, there are some sterling images of good patient care showing up on film. But, unfortunately, they are the exception.

The obvious defects are the most basic of patient care skills — failure to use a backboard, failure to apply a cervical collar, improper CPR technique, incorrect methods for administering oxygen. The people committing these errors are not *bad* people, and those who trained them probably were not *bad* teachers. But the photos tell us that something *bad* has happened. It shouldn't be necessary to go through 20 or 30 photos of emergency action before finding one that's fit to publish.

Probably, people who are attracted to prehospital care have a little actor in them. Nearly every call is a stressful performance, and nearly every performance has an audience. Those who prefer to perform in private usually don't last long in EMS.

Every actor knows that every performance will be reviewed critically. There will always be people in the audience who can tell a good performance from a poor one. Increasingly, the North American public is able to distinguish good prehospital care from mediocre. Forty-million Americans have been trained in CPR; many of them can spot incorrect techniques.

As we train this year's crop of about 100,000 new EMTs, let's try to impress upon them that they will be actors on a stage once they get out on the street. They will be performing for a critical audience — many of whom know something about good patient care. Let's remind them that photographers will catch some of their performances, and that the photographic image of sloppy care cannot be explained away.

At the very least, let's remind ourselves and our trainees that grieving family, friends and neighbors (and passersby on a crowded interstate) cannot share our humor or the back-slapping of old pals who happen to meet at the scene of an emergency. In virtually every emergency, there are numerous "victims" (some are only bystanders), and we need to perform as professionals before all of them.

Friday the 13th

I've never been superstitious. Black cats have always been welcome across my path. If the shortest route goes under a ladder, so be it. A broken mirror has never been cause for alarm. But that was prior to last July 13th (a Friday).

The first hint of trouble was a power outage while I was operating a computer at the office. I'm still not sure what was lost when the microchip went into asystole. Later, my wife called to report that our sale of some property back east had collapsed on the last day of escrow.

About noon, I decided a workout at the gym would be preferable to lunch (and might even change my luck). As I backed my aged Volvo out of its space in the parking lot, reverse gear and third gear somehow got a ball bearing between them — an event accompanied by great gnashing and transmission trauma. A little later, I learned that my youngest son had just bought a motorcycle. The day was significant for other reasons. A job I'd been preparing myself for during the past 20 years was open. It was the top management position in a big west coast fire department that handles about 100,000 EMS calls a year. I had filed an application, but the personnel bureaucracy wouldn't let me take the exam. I had appealed their decision and, if the appeal was to be successful, I would hear from them on Friday, the 13th, at the latest. They never called. Oh, well. What's 20 years?

After dinner, with a full moon on the horizon, I drove back to the *JEMS* office (in second gear). My wife gathered a young niece and nephew into her new station wagon and headed for the beach. She parked the car next to the coastal road in Del Mar and took the kids across the beach to walk at the water's edge.

Meanwhile, Hugh Stewart Muncie, age 22, was drunk and driving his '66 Mustang at a high rate of speed along the coastal road. He swerved to pass another car and struck the raised center road divider, ricocheted to the opposite side of the road, struck an asphalt berm and became airborne. The flying Mustang bounced on its side atop my wife's new car, finally ending up on its wheels a car length off the road.

Hugh Stewart Muncie was on the verge of death, bleeding internally from a ruptured spleen and other injuries. His 26-year-old male passenger had been thrown from the car and suffered equally serious injuries. Both young men were taken by paramedics to a trauma center. Surgeons worked to save their lives within the Golden Hour.

Mr. Muncie will live to drive again. Will he again drive while drunk? Will he again endanger my family and others with severely antisocial behavior? Will he feel any debt or obligation to the community that created the trauma system that saved his life? A bumper strip on his wrecked car announced that he is a musician. Will he write a song about the selfish and irresponsible compulsion to drink and drive a car?

Aside from superstition, July 13th shared with me another view of trauma care. If Mr. Muncie had succeeded in killing or injuring my family, I wouldn't be all that thrilled with the trauma care system that saved his life — that is, unless he learns from his experience, corrects his behavior, and works diligently to prevent others from acting as he did.

Through all the debates over trauma care, we've heard lots of talk about our obligation to take care of trauma victims. But what about those trauma victims who cause their own trauma and hurt others in the process? Don't they have some obligations?

If I were the judge who sentences Hugh Stewart Muncie, I would attach some special conditions to his parole — after the jail term. I would require him to spend about 52 Friday nights doing janitorial work in a busy trauma center. One who mops up the blood of drunk drivers and their victims just might get the message.

The Spectator

Under an exchange arrangement, *JEMS* receives most of the hundred or so EMS bulletins, newsletters and magazines that are published in the U.S. And we read them — it helps us to keep our finger on what's happening in our field. Recently, the editorial in one of those publications dealt with the public's magnetic attraction to gore and death.

I remember reading it for the first time. The editor was describing a scene where there were mutliple fatalities and hundreds of curious spectators, some with their children, pressing for a view of the carnage. The editor was offended by it all and urged readers to protect the privacy of victims' families as much as possible.

Those written comments brought back some long-buried memories: a small plane that fell from the sky into a residential neighborhood on a Sunday afternoon; a multiple homicide in a crowded apartment house. Numerous fires that snuffed out numerous lives. Countless auto accidents with gruesome injuries or deaths. And always the spectators, ever pressing forward to get a better look.

We were conditioned to be angry at the spectators, to shout at them and try to make them feel like "low life." After all, what kind of people would rush to the scene just to look at burnt bodies, or mangled limbs, or blood? "What's the matter with you people? Get the hell outta here!" Some of them would slink away. Others would shout back with references to our ancestry.

A few weeks ago, this topic came up while visiting with a friend who is not a rescuer. His reaction flew in the face of more than 20 years of conditioning: "As one of those lay people who can't resist trying to see what's going on at an accident (if I can stay out of the way), I'm always put off by the attitude of some rescue workers that 'rubber neckers' are just one shade better than necrophiliacs."

It threw me off balance. I had never thought of this friend as one of those strange faceless people who crowd around the scene of an emergency. In fact, I don't think I'd ever met one of them before. And he's really a nice guy! My mind flashed with the question of how he'd react if I shouted for him to "Get outta here!"

He continued: "I was at the beach the other day when a near-drowning took place. Obviously, people milled around to see what was going on as the lifeguards worked on the guy. But wouldn't it be pretty *un*natural if people were so disinterested that they sat on their beach towels and continued talking about what's for dinner, while a life-and-death drama took place within yards of them?"

He had a point. If I had been there, I would have been in the middle of the emergency. I would have justified running to the scene by telling myself that I might know what to do. But if the lifeguards were already there, would

I leave? If not, how much of the compulsion to stick around would be plain and simple curiosity? If the lifeguards told me to "Get outta here," how would I react?

My friend continued, "I guess what I'm trying to say is, don't get mad at a dog that licks its genitals in public, and don't get mad at people who can't resist trying to see what all the fuss is about — it's part of their nature. You don't cope with an 'uncivilized' dog that is ruining your appetite by kicking him in the side. You understand it's the nature of the beast, no matter how distasteful, and gently (but forcefully) remove him from your view."

My friend has a vivid way of describing things. He also presents some tough questions. For example: "Isn't being part of the action one reason a lot of people get into fire, police or rescue work in the first place?" While I was still thinking about the question, he answered it, "Lay people have a natural desire to be on the inside too. Sure, they can be obnoxious and get in your way. But if they do get in your way, just remove them; don't make moral judgments about how sick they all are, and then let that attitude creep into your methods of dispersal."

A few days after that conversation, I was traveling and happened onto the remnants of a multiple vehicle collision. I stopped, justifying my behavior as a valid journalistic interest. All the victims had been removed but the mangled vehicles were spattered with blood. A crowd of people stood around watching as the tow trucks prepared to disentangle the wrecked cars. I looked at the faces in the crowd; they looked like regular people.

Out in the street, several firefighters and a police officer were laughing about something one of them had said. The lady standing next to me reacted: "That's disgusting! All those people killed and hurt, and they're out there laughing." She turned and walked away.

I wanted to say, "But lady, they see this sort of thing all the time." Then the irony of it all hit me. She had come to the scene out of curiosity — a natural response. She had endured the ugly visions of twisted metal, broken bodies and blood. But she was driven away by the sight of an *un*-natural response — rescuers who had become calloused and indifferent to their human environment.

I've done it. Probably, you have too. And possibly we deserve as much criticism as we've heaped on those "rubber neckers" over the years.

Front-Page Gore

Francis L. Fears got his picture in the paper one day in August. He was on the cover of the Sunday edition of the Richardson (Texas) *Daily News*. It was his last photograph, but it wasn't the way he would want to be remembered.

In the photo, Fears was on his back, spread-eagled on a grassy field. His shirt had been ripped open and his trousers had been pulled down to his knees. A tube was taped to his gaping mouth, and the very efficient arm and plunger of a mechanical CPR device was over his chest. EKG leads were attached to Mr. Fears in all the right places and an intense young paramedic straddled him with defribrillator paddles gripped by muscular arms. In the foreground, a paramedic prepared another IV; in the background, a third paramedic appeared to be checking for blood pressure.

It was a graphic illustration of prehospital emergency care at its best. It appeared to be a textbook version of treating cardiac arrest on the street. It might even serve a useful purpose in training other paramedics. But it was a terrible indignity to Mr. Fears and his family, displayed as it was for public consumption on the front page of a daily newspaper.

"I am angered, shocked and horrified beyond words that your paper would print a photograph of this nature. This is in my opinion another example of irresponsible journalism," wrote one reader to the editor of the *Daily News*. "I am absolutely incredulous at the lack of human compassion displayed by this disrespectful act. Did it not cross your minds that a family member, friend or fellow employee of this unfortunate victim might see the photograph and become upset?"

Another reader wrote: "The picture of the paramedics trying to revive Mr. Fears was absolutely disgusting! I only hope that this poor man's family did not see this photograph. Can you imagine how they will feel seeing their husband, father or son lying stripped about half naked on the ground?" she asked. "I realize what you must have meant in publishing this photo and the work the paramedics do is one that should not go unnoticed, but must it be displayed in such an untactful manner?"

Another lady was similarly upset. "I think the (*Daily News*) owes the family of (Mr. Fears) an apology. You violated his right to privacy at a time when he was unable to defend the right."

One angry reader ordered the paper to cancel his subscription. "The photograph of the dying man was really a cheap shot. You took the last moments of a man's life and turned them into an attention grabber. The man in the picture is beyond caring, but I suspect you may have caused his family enormous additional pain."

People in most professions tend to look forward to the

ultimate challenge. Most paramedics get energized by the periodic "full arrest" situation, especially if they are successful. Even though prevention is supposed to be the first priority for firefighters, most of them derive professional satisfaction from attacking the fully involved structure fire. Similarly, news photographers look for the most exciting action and human drama situations to focus on. And publishers strive for the opportunity to generate more subscriber and ad revenue by beating the competition to eye-catching stories and photos.

The problem with all this "ultimate challenge" stuff is keeping it in perspective. We've known some paramedics who consider anything but a full arrest case to be a "garbage call." We know lots of firefighters who ignore the responsibility to fire prevention while they verbally re-fight old fires and look forward to the next "big one." Francis Fears was the victim of a newspaper's zeal to put in print the ultimate human drama. A photograph with a different angle would have done the job, while sparing the indignity.

Rich Adams, a Maryland EMT who serves as editorial director for a Washington TV station, lectures that EMS services need to stay in close touch with their local press. What would a news photographer hear if he dropped by our respective stations for an occasional cup of coffee? Would we inadvertently blow his perspective of our business by offering him endless stories about the ultimate challenges? Or would we balance the discussion by offering some humane views on the patient's need for privacy and dignity, or the family's grief in the aftermath of a sudden and unexpected death?

If your local news people have a tendency to zero in on the gore (at the expense of all else), why not invite them over to visit? Maybe you could share a copy of this column, especially the letters to the editor of the Richardson *Daily News*. The old adage that controversy sells newspapers has its limits. There can be no honor nor satisfaction in promoting sales and revenue through the infliction of unnecessary emotional pain and indignity.

The Underclass Crisis

There's an issue that threatens more than a decade of progress in EMS and suggests a distressing future. For lack of a better term, we've been referring to it as the growth of the EMS underclass.

The problem involves the difference between big numbers and individual attitudes. The big numbers tell us there is a currently licensed or certified EMT for every 476 men, women and children in the U.S. But our reading of attitudes during the past years tells us that doesn't mean very much. With increasing frequency, we've encountered an anti-training, anti-improvement, anti-responsibility attitude among some people who carry cards and wear patches that suggest they're worthy and capable of holding others' lives in their hands.

"This is a bunch of crap," one EMT told us as he begrudgingly endured a 40-hour refresher course. He grumbled that he had learned it all before and didn't need to be exposed to the same information or subjected to another test.

"Our members are too busy tryin' to earn a living and don't have time to take a CPR course," a volunteer told us. (They have a beautiful white-and-orange ambulance, operated by people who haven't even been trained in the most basic of emergency care techniques.) A fire chief told us he thought the EMT course tried to teach his people more than they needed to know.

The EMS training director in one of our larger states reported to us that as many as 50 percent of his state's EMTs are failing to recertify. But they're still running on ambulance calls. We could go on and on listing the danger signs. It's sufficient to note that the next major crisis in EMS is already here.

In many states, legislation has been enacted to require that ambulances are staffed by properly trained and certified personnel. But laws don't enforce themselves; and EMS officials in most states lack the will, or the staff or the political clout to enforce their own laws. Even if the laws were strictly enforced, the enforcement campaign would not produce a caring attitude in the offenders. No law can remedy the dangerous attitude that one has no responsibility to the public. No legislation can open the closed minds of people who feel they already know everything they want to know.

In exploring this topic, we've considered many factors which may be feeding the growth of the EMS underclass, including EMT training. As it's become institutionalized in the educational network, has EMT training become simply a variation of welding, or auto mechanics, or sheetmetal working? Does every EMT instructor convey the essence of professionalism that would inspire EMT trainees to recognize and actively pursue their responsibility to the patient?

Speaking of education, could it be that the problem relates to the fact that one in five Americans is functionally illiterate (including some with high school diplomas)? How many of those who oppose training or testing actually are presenting a smoke screen against the fact that they are unable to read or write adequately? We think it's significant that less than four percent of all EMTs belong to their national association, less than eight percent ever attend an EMS educational conference, and only about 10 percent subscribe to a professional journal.

One of our readers, Mark Blum, suggested that the goals of continuing education programs need to be reassessed, so good EMTs aren't "thrown out with the wash." Despite our intense interest in the topic, we haven't been able to formulate any conclusions. We've shared our concern about the EMS underclass with knowledgeable people throughout the country, and they have validated our concerns. It's a crisis, and it's here and now.

The Making of a Hero

One of the fire service publications has an annual program of awards for acts of heroism or community service. After they had their annual awards, several of our readers suggested that *JEMS* do something like it for EMS people. While we were pondering the idea (how to do it fairly, how not to miss deserving people, whether such a program would contribute to the quality of emergency care), Associate Editor Thom Dick shared with me another view of heroism.

Not long ago, a California police agency received a report of "shots fired" in a mobile home park. Eventually, three people died and two others were injured, including a sheriff's captain who went to the door of the gunman's mobile home. A .22 caliber bullet fired by the 57-year-old resident lodged in the captain's neck near his carotid artery.

A sheriff's deputy received instant acclaim for dragging the captain to cover, thus saving his life. The county sheriff talked of nominating the female deputy to receive civic awards for her reported actions. For three days, the public recognized her as a heroine.

But the inside story went like this: The sheriff's captain, discovering his injury, never lost consciousness. "I'm shot! I'm shot!," he said, as he ran back to his patrol car and laid down on the ground. A third deputy frantically motioned to a waiting paramedic crew, directing them into the line of fire.

Without hesitation, the paramedics and their EMT partner ran to the side of the injured police officer. He was then placed on a cot, pulled out of the danger area, placed in an ambulance, treated by the paramedics, and then transported to the nearest hospital.

Meanwhile, at the scene of the emergency, a second paramedic unit was standing by. A call came across the radio to respond to the aid of an unconscious diabetic lying in a restaurant less than a block away. The paramedics took the call begrudgingly. "Send an EMT unit," one of them protested. "We want to stay where the action is."

The drama of the shooting emergency went on. Newsmen pushed and shoved, jabbing rescuers with cameras and mikes, and competing with hundreds of spectators for a look at what was going on.

In homes throughout the region, people were tuned in to the six o'clock news. "Our helicopter is at the scene at this moment," announced one newscaster, "but we're keeping our spotlights off because we want to protect the lives of the SWAT team members."

Next morning, the team of paramedics who had rescued the sheriff's captain were going off duty. The relief crew questioned them about the shooting incident. The guys modestly described their actions and credited one another for the apparent bravery. None could remember seeing the female deputy who had been the focus of the news broadcasts. When asked about her, they just shrugged their shoulders.

Later, when the press finally caught up with the female deputy, she said she didn't remember rescuing her colleague. The story just sort of died.

As it turned out, the captain's wound wasn't serious, and he wasn't shot again as he lay on the ground, or as he was carried away. Nor were the rescuers who removed him from danger. A year from now, the police officer will have forgotten the paramedics' names: in fact, he may never have heard them at all.

Meanwhile, an EMT arrives at a convalescent home with her partner to transfer an old woman to a hospital. Before moving her, the crew notices that the woman is grossly incontinent of feces. The nurses are "too busy" to clean her up. The woman hides her face in shame.

The EMT reassures the woman and proceeds to clean her up. There is nothing in the EMT's job description that says she's required to do this, but she does it. There are no TV cameras around. There are no bullets flying. There are no paramedics.

"There," she says, finished, and the old woman reaches for her hand in thanks.

The EMT's name is Ruth Ann McGuire. She is gentle and soft-spoken. There are many like her. Their names and their kindnesses have never been published. They are the greatest heroes of all. Obviously, there will never be enough pages in any publication to include appropriate awards or recognition for all of them.

4

Motivation and Leadership

So You Want to be an EMS Leader

My young friend has been hungry for a bigger piece of the action. He's got a reasonable education under his belt. He's proven himself as an EMT and paramedic. He moved far from home to take his first job in EMS administration. It gave him a chance to adapt from the unknown challenges of the street to the more predictable and tedious challenges of a desk. But those challenges became routine before long and he started looking for the next rung on his career ladder.

He would call me every month or so. Did I know of any jobs that might be opening up? Occasionally, I would be able to share some scuttlebutt about a new position, or one that was vacated (usually because the prior occupant got fired). My friend would follow up with a resume and a letter.

I've always enjoyed the opportunity to help bright young people meet their occupational or professional goals. Sometimes as an employer, other times as a reference, I've been able to maneuver some of these friends into challenging new jobs — as regional EMS project directors, county ambulance service managers, or state EMS directors. About half the time, I've been very proud of their performances in new and important positions. The rest of the time, I've been disappointed — or embarrassed.

I feel an embarrassment coming on. My hungry young friend finally got a chance to escape from his mundane desk in Podunk. He landed an impressive EMS administration job with an impressive title in a big and important place. Maybe he was hungry too long. For, when he finally got a sniff of real authority, it began to intoxicate him.

Soon, the impressive job wasn't impressive enough. With all the finesse of a dump truck, he began to seek more power. Even the impressive title wasn't impressive enough. He arranged for a new title which possessed greater regal trappings.

In his quest for approval and recognition my friend attracted the opposite reaction. His "power grabs" produced a flurry of sarcastic jokes and humorous imitations. Not to his face, of course. As this was happening, my friend displayed his greatest shortcoming. He was insensitive to the mood surrounding him. He really thought he was pulling it off. In reality, he had become totally ineffective; nobody could take him seriously.

The biggest mistake, however, was the persistent compulsion to tell locals "how we did it in ____________________." The locals pretended to be interested, face-to-face. Behind his back, they crucified him.

I'm not sure how my friend got the message. But he escaped with a modicum of his dignity. He's got another job now (he didn't ask for my help this time). And, I'm sorry to report, he's making all the same mistakes. I suspect he'll be completely removed from the EMS field in a year or two.

I've thought about calling my friend and giving him some "fatherly" advice. But it's not easy to tell someone that they're making a fool of themselves. Maybe he'll read this and figure out that he's the subject matter. But I doubt it. Ego trips most often occur in tunnels.

So *you* want to be an EMS leader someday? If your desire is strong enough, and you have a reasonable degree of talent, you'll probably make it. I hope you'll save yourself a lot of grief and heed the sorry experience of many of your predecessors.

Be aware that you'll be trying to lead people who aren't easily impressed. They've seen life at its most miserable and death at its most gruesome. When you're decorating your new office, put all of your diplomas and awards in the closet. When people start to address you as "Chief" or "Director" or "Mister," insist that they call you by your first name.

No matter where you've come from, no matter what you did while there, don't mention it unless asked specifically (and then mention the bad along with the good). The universal turn-off in EMS is the guy who's forever telling "how we did it in ____________________." If things were so good, why did you leave?

Be sensitive to progress that's already been made in your new bailiwick. My friend has been marching through his new domain, proclaiming that the local continuing education program is a joke. If he'd spent a little time asking questions, and *listening*, he'd have learned that the program is really quite good. It has been constructed with the hard work of some talented people who now look forward to the downfall of my young friend.

I'm planning to take a vacation from my role as EMS matchmaker — the mistakes always haunt me. And maybe no help is really needed for those who are sincerely interested in improving patient care and can match their talent and ambition with a basic respect for their fellow workers. Jobs always seem to open up for them, anyway.

A Call for Participative Management

As a kid, growing up in L.A., I was impressed by a man named Bill Parker, and the peerless organization he crafted from the debris of earlier scandal and corruption. Parker was chief of police, and his life and obsession (LAPD) in many ways became an extension of his own personality. In those days, LAPD officers bristled with pride and loyalty to the organization, projecting an esprit de corps comparable to a victorious battalion of Marines.

Bill Parker died of a ruptured aneurism several years ago. And many of the social and political changes since his death have affected the organization he coerced into excellence. It's a different world, and it's a different LAPD.

For example, the loyalty of the troops and middle managers has turned to deep distrust of the top brass. According to a recent study, LAPD employees feel that human needs such as support, opportunity

---

NOTE: This appeared in JEMS *in March, 1982.*

for development, forgiveness, trust, openness and honesty, all seem to come second to procedures, systems and technology.

In a fascinating display of leadership and courage, current Police Chief Daryl Gates ordered the study, and then ordered the results to be distributed throughout the department — including critiques of his own leadership. Further, he dispatched a letter to all personnel reaffirming his commitment to make LAPD "a place where everybody likes to come to work." According to the letter, he is working on ways to bring field officers into the department's decision-making process.

The study included anonymous surveys and personal interviews of department officials, from captains to deputy chiefs. The report quoted one as saying, "We carry on in an atmosphere where we do very little for our employees but do a great deal to them." "None of us listen or know how to listen very well," said another. Still another, suggesting the existence of a "seige mentality," said, ". . . we are not open to good communication from inside or outside." According to one respondent, "There is very little room for healthy disagreement in the police department."

One of the LAPD officials' comments easily might have been directed to the management atmosphere of many EMS agencies: "Our training has produced managers and supervisors who are too mechanical — system- and task-oriented — rather than people oriented. As a result, our people want a shopping list and guidelines rather than a problem or a challenge. If you don't know how to manage people well, then you adopt a management philosophy which relates to things."

If Bill Parker had lived long enough, he might have faced the same problems Daryl Gates is dealing with. As Gates points out, his leadership is compromised by such factors as an unsupportive mayor, five consecutive years of city council budget cutbacks, critical media coverage and a troublesome police union. He says this collection of influences has "disintegrated the family attitude in the department."

It seems to me that the apparent problems at LAPD are more than a little familiar to EMS people, career and volunteer alike. We hear lots of griping about EMS organizations where there is little room for healthy disagreement. We hear about EMS organizations where the leadership does little for members or employees, but plenty to them. We see the compulsion to issue shopping lists and guidelines (often in the form of overly detailed "protocols"), rather than accept problems and the challenge of solving them. And we hear career EMS people commenting on how much they *don't* like to go to work.

Bill Parker managed his organization in simpler times: he probably would never have permitted the critical assessment Daryl Gates asked for and got. But if Gates follows through on his stated intention to humanize LAPD, he may prove himself as right for the times as Bill Parker was. In the meantime, wouldn't it be encouraging to see more fire chiefs and EMS managers with the courage to engage in participative management?

There's no guarantee that Gates' efforts to improve morale will work. According to my sources, the cynicism in the ranks is deep and epidemic. But like many of the fire chiefs and EMS managers I know, Daryl Gates has no choice. (The difference is that *he* understands he's got no choice.) If he fails to restore the family atmosphere by making people more important than things, the department will explode, and leave his career in the rubble. If his best efforts fail, at least he'll be able to peer from the rubble with his pride intact. Personally, I hope he succeeds. The lessons of his success will become the stuff of management textbooks, and humanizing the police-fire-EMS working environment might even become a fad.

POSTSCRIPT: Almost five years later, I tried to check on Chief Gates' progress. After talking to people in and around the organization, I came to a sad conclusion: the cynicism and distrust in the ranks is as bad as ever. Street cops don't feel they have a piece of the department's decision-making process. They feel that there is no tolerance within the department for healthy disagreement. The ones I talked to don't even remember the 1982 study and report.

When I called police headquarters and tried to get some assessments from the brass, the real problem came into focus. LAPD, like most of today's organizations, has a shortage of candor and coverage at the middle management level. They remember the 1982 study alright, but nobody was willing to comment on the impact or results. "Do you think communications within the organization are better, worse or about the same?" I asked. Inevitably, that question got my call transferred to someone else (I gave up before finding anyone with enough guts to offer an opinion).

On the positive side, Daryl Gates can be proud that he took the first big, bold step toward participative management. Even if the desired results are hard to find, the eye of the average citizen still sees LAPD as the best looking, best trained, most incorruptible of the big city police departments.

Time of the Parenthesis

In his best-selling book, *Megatrends: Ten New Directions Transforming Our Lives*, author John Naisbitt referred to our period of history as the "time of the parenthesis — a time between eras." It's important to examine some of the more important implications of being between eras in the world of emergency medical services.

The biggest implication surely is the uncertainty of it all. At every turn, we are seeing and hearing that much of what we learned and did in the past won't be applicable in the future. Even the ways we related to other people in the past may not work in the present or the future.

Naisbitt refers to this time between eras as "great and yeasty, filled with opportunity." He suggests that those who can handle the ambiguity of this in-between period and anticipate the new era will be a quantum leap ahead of those who hold on to old ideas and practices. In fact, he says, we can learn to make uncertainty our friend and we can achieve much more than in stable times.

For the first time since best-seller lists were invented, the books at the top of those lists are about business, the future, the economy, and how to manage organizations. Clearly, people who buy books are looking for guidance in this uncertain time between eras. We've seen evidence that many of the leaders in EMS are reading those books — trying to get a vision of the road ahead.

Victims of sudden and unexpected illness or injury deserve effective prehospital care and transportation, delivered by well-trained, motivated and properly equipped personnel. Quality assurance can be achieved in one of two ways. Either do it yourself (so you'll know it gets done right), or control and influence the behavior of others so that they will do it right. Instructors, field supervisors, medical directors, lieutenants, captains, chiefs and EMS officials all must use the second alternative. They are unable to care for every patient themselves, so they must control and influence the behavior of others. What's the best way to do that in the era of megatrends?

Naisbitt wrote that "we have extraordinary leverage and influence — individually, professionally, and institutionally — if we can only get a clear sense, a clear conception, a clear vision, of the road ahead." It's our opinion that the road ahead is far different than the road behind. When it comes to controlling and influencing the performance and behavior of others, those who continue to use the old road map will be lost.

Excessive regulation, draconian edicts and top-down management were common techniques for control in the era past. The style and content of control often depended on the background or bias of the person or persons currently holding the power. In EMS, there were distinct differences in the control and influence of systems if those in power had an orientation to nursing, surgery, emergency medicine, public health or fire protection. Often, power was shared only with those who fit into the reigning category.

Our vision of the road ahead is clear. Power will be shared with all who have some responsibility to perform. People will refuse to be "managed" but will hunger for leadership. Top-down assertion of control will give way to participative governance. The regulatory role of government will diminish. Volumes of regulations will be replaced by value statements developed by consensus. Individual responsibility and peer review will thrive in the place of semi-judicial bureaucratic discipline.

There is much to be relinquished by some and much to be gained by others — including those we serve. The fact that change will occur is a clear sign that the road ahead will be difficult. But change we must. We are in the time between eras; to avoid or resist adaptation is to become a relic of the past.

For those who depend on rank or position to control or influence the behavior of others, these are troubling times. Those who presume that the letter of the law automatically commands the respect and compliance of the governed apparently have not heard of tax evasion, the 55 mph speed limit, or illegal drugs.

As we all continue our quest for the best in emergency medical care, some may grieve the passing of old times, beliefs and practices. We are more inclined to embrace the expression of John Naisbitt: "My God, what a fantastic time to be alive!"

A Return to Competence

The $200 tune-up turned our year-old car into a pinging, lurching, coughing, dying pile of iron. The brand-new house revealed its qualities as the winter winds whistled through misfit windows. The kids' Christmas toys were inoperable before January arrived. The street repair crew fixed a pothole — but left a mound of asphalt to rattle the teeth of every driver who passes over it.

For several years, we've been watching competence and reliability fade from memory. As our nation's economic underpinnings have switched from an industrial base to a variety of "service industries," satisfactory service (of any kind) has become an endangered species.

Whatever happened to the people who made our nation the greatest in the world? What became of the proud craftsmen whose products now bring inflated prices at antique auctions?

Our apparent national slide into mediocrity probably has a multitude of causes. We would hang some of the blame on so-called consumer advocates who would have us believe that quality, competence and safe products can be achieved by legislation and regulatory agencies. A whole generation now believes that someone in a position of authority is going to protect them from cradle to grave.

Seldom mentioned in the great discussions of "industrial productivity" is the fact that a significant population of American workers are *stoned*. A noon-time walk along Wall Street in New York reveals clerical types toking joints before returning to the tedium of their jobs. A murder in an auto assembly plant reveals the existence of a complex drug-dealing network. Insiders allege that increased costs and reduced quality in film and television are due to an epidemic of drug use in the industry.

No other society in the history of mankind has had so many choices, so much discretionary income, so much freedom. Our economic plenty seems to have made us a "throw-away" society, never concerned about tomorrow nor the long-term costs of today's good life. Competence and reliability have suffered greatly in this environment. Can we return to competence and reliability without eroding our basic freedom? That may be the biggest question and challenge of our times.

There seems to be a growing desire among North Americans to return to the greatness which we have taken for granted. But a society which is wallowing in the refuse of easy times needs an example to follow. Some individual or group must lead the way. The first steps must be taken by people who try very hard to be what they say they are, people who are never quite satisfied that they are doing their jobs as well as they might be done. We think there are many examples among North America's EMS workers.

We think most EMS people are setting such an example for our society. Surely, there are EMTs, nurses and doctors who are faking it — content that some long-ago training course adequately prepared them for competent patient care. But the majority of us scoff at these pretenders. We refuse to follow their mediocre examples. We flock to continuing education courses and seek out better ways to serve people in need.

In the age of competence, the master carpenter or the skilled mason was fiercely proud of his finished product. We've watched a lot of EMS people perform their craft in recent years and we've noted that many of them are fiercely proud of what they can do, even when they are unable to make the patient whole again. At least they know they did their best — they held back nothing in their efforts to serve with competence. A few months ago, a public health administrator told us that "paramedics irritate the hell out of me; they are so damned self-righteous." Our response: "If they are as good as they should be, they have a right to be self-righteous."

We think EMS, particularly *pre*hospital care, holds promise as a pace-setter in the return to competence and reliability in our North American culture. If EMS proves that there is something that can be relied upon, some service that will live up to public expectations, it will be because individual EMS workers will have lived up to their personal responsibility to themselves and their patients. The motivation to be as good as we should be must come from within. It cannot be produced by a government regulation. Although training and continuing education are important, it is the individual's commitment to learning that will make the difference. In the end, if competence and reliability generates "self-righteousness," we will welcome it as a vast improvement over fakery and sloppiness.

Rumor Has It . . .

Switch on the television and witness a marvel of information transfer. Live reports by commentators in Moscow, Tokyo and New York race around the globe in a split second to be delivered to our homes with color and clarity. Where Marco Polo devoted many years in traveling to foreign lands, electronic information now can be transmitted across those same distances in little more than the span of a heartbeat.

Here at home a few years ago, a chewing gum manufacturer suffered major losses when pre-teen kids across the nation spread the rumor that the gum was made of spider eggs. More recently, a soap manufacturer was victimized by a rumor that spread across the country like a firestorm. According to the rumor, the company's long-time trademark had some link to satanic worship. Actress Jane Fonda recently found it necessary to appear on news broadcasts to disprove the widespread rumor that she had suffered a heart attack.

The revolution of electronic information was predicted and discussed at length in past years. Some felt it would greatly enhance the human condition by delivering us from rumor through instant access to facts. They didn't anticipate the probability that rumor, while less efficient and often totally inaccurate, would remain a preferred method of communicating.

The tenacity (and possible growth) of rumor as a means of communicating affects us all in the field of EMS. In many cases where states have made changes in EMT or paramedic training or testing, rumors have run rampant in the field about what those changes will be and how they will affect one group or another. In those places where new designs for ambulance service have been proposed, unfounded rumors about the consequences have caused near-panic among employees of the existing services in that locale.

Probably the most common topic of rumor in EMS is that of lawsuits, both real and imagined. Despite abundant published material on the topic, misinformation seems to travel the grapevine with efficiency that rivals the electronic networks.

There are a couple of things that bother us about rumors and those who go out of their way to spread them. Inevitably, the information they convey is negative. Have you ever heard a rumor that was upbeat and promising, that made you feel better? Secondly, the whole time-consuming process of hearing, thinking about, discussing and passing on rumors detracts from what we should be concentrating on — the best possible patient care we can provide.

The next time someone carries a rumor to you, it might be interesting to start your own personal rumor log. Jot down the date, the basic message and who told it, and then wait to see whether it comes true. Keep track of each rumor for a year or more. Eventually, we suspect your rumor log will reveal the same person or people as chronic purveyors of bum information.

It would be easy to blame the "street people" of EMS — those who deliver prehospital care on the street — for the injudicious spreading of inaccurate information. But we think equal blame must be shared by those in control. Employers who don't communicate with employees should expect active minds to speculate and spread speculation. The EMS officials should recognize the need for constant contact and communication — in the field — with those they are supposed to motivate and control.

For the chronic rumor-mongers, we offer another thought. As our wonderful nation is being whipped in so many ways in so many corners of the globe, it's important for all of us to contribute to efficiency and excellence. The economic and social machine of North America is retarded every time human effort and energy is detoured by misinformation. Spreading rumors could be considered anti-American. To the extent that it detracts us from our roles as emergency care providers, it could be downright life-threatening.

Ask an EMT

A few weeks ago, an EMT and his partner found themselves across a desk from an EMS administrator. They had requested the meeting. They wanted to explain why some of the administrator's policies, guidelines and protocols actually had a negative effect on patient care.

They didn't make much headway. In the process of gaining little bits of understanding and change, they had to do a lot of explaining. They found themselves in a defensive position. The administrator, after all, was an "EMS expert" (based on formal education and official position). On the other hand, this "expert" had never been in an ambulance.

We know lots of EMS administrators who've "done it on the street," so to speak. Some of them continue to pull ambulance duty whenever possible, just to keep some balance between the realities of patient care and the lofty policies, guidelines and protocols.

Many others, however, perform their administrative

tasks in a vacuum of real-world patient care experience. It's like a chief pilot who's never flown, or a school administrator who's never taught. A public health official may be able to run a rodent control program without ever touching a rat, or an immunization program without ever contracting the disease. But we've seldom seen an administrator who could competently control the activities of EMTs without at least being with them in action.

We have a suggestion for those who may fit the description. Spend some time riding with your EMTs. Not with your paramedics, or your EMT brother-in-law and his partner. Spend some time with the newest crew in your system — and not just from nine to five. Do it all day and all night. If they can do it, so can you (but if you *can't*, maybe they can't either).

You've got a computer, you say? It tells you all you need to know about the system? Believe us, all that computerized information about response times and call loads will take on a new dimension if you'll ride with your crews routinely, on a scheduled basis — and you should.

You should be looking in cabinets, slamming doors and riding on ambulance cots. What kind of ride do your units give to patients with major fractures? You should be trying out some of that budget equipment; does it do what it's supposed to? Are your blankets really warm enough? For that matter, how about your crews' jackets? How do the dispatchers treat your EMTs?

You've read all about how EMS has improved in the last ten years? You should check behind the doors of your town's convalescent homes. You'll find that if your EMTs ask too many questions or (God forbid) get caught taking vital signs, some nurse is likely to take their names and make a phone call. Next time she needs an ambulance, she'll call an agency that's less "trouble."

Most nurses who *have* any important information usually seal it in an envelope. Your job, as an EMT, is to "just take this patient to the hospital," and you'll know better than to open that envelope.

The emergency nurses and physicians in your area probably pay close attention when your paramedic crews call them on the radio. But notice what happens when one of your EMT crews makes a complete, concise report. Chances are, a clerk will take the information, condense it a little, write it on a piece of scratch paper, and place it where it won't be found for a few hours.

While you're at it, notice what most emergency physicians think of your EMTs' splinting efforts (as they remove equipment at random, without listening to information about mechanisms of injury). If you happen to see a nurse or physician do something you're sure is wrong, forget about it. That's what your EMTs do; they don't stand a chance of keeping their jobs otherwise, and they know it.

Probably, you've instructed your EMTs to take acute patients to the closest hospital equipped and staffed to handle their problems. But have you told them what to do when the patient insists on going to the "wrong" hospital? You need to experience *that* conflict as it's happening, on the street.

One more thing. When you ride with your EMTs, don't tell the communications center that you're aboard. Dress in an EMT's uniform. Get yourself an EMT's nametag. Work, eat and sleep like an EMT. Humiliating? Hard work? Maybe so, but no matter how important you think you are, it's your job to know what kind of service your system is providing.

Better than anybody else in the system, your basic life support EMTs know how the system's performing. They make contact with almost *all* the patients, even when the paramedics are called as well.

Maybe none of these problems apply to your system. Maybe they all do, and more besides. The fact is, if you don't put yourself into a position to find out, you can't know for sure. But maybe your successor will.

POSTSCRIPT: Thanks to Thom Dick, JEMS *Associate Editor, who inspired (and provided much of the content of) this article after he had worked undercover as a basic EMT.*

Values versus Regulations

The big question in EMS right now, and in fact in every profession and business in this country, is deceivingly simple: "what is the best way to control and influence the behavior of others?"

If you've been around a while, you might think the answer is straightforward. Set minimum standards, provide a book of regulations, and discipline those who don't toe the line. If you stay with me through this essay, I'll show you why that answer doesn't work anymore.

First, let me introduce you to Eugene and Bonnie. Eugene is an EMT and Bonnie is an emergency nurse. Bonnie likes cocaine. She likes it a lot. Bonnie also likes Eugene. She doesn't like Eugene a lot, but she pretends she does because Eugene always seems to have cocaine or knows where to get it.

Bonnie and Eugene go to lots of parties. Sometimes, they see Albert at parties. He's an emergency physician and he does drugs too. He's pretty discrete about it, but Bonnie can always tell when Albert is high, even when he's working.

Bonnie and Eugene and Albert and many of their friends know that getting caught in possession of or under the influence of drugs would cost them their licenses or certificates, not to mention their jobs. That risk doesn't seem to affect them; they continue to do drugs and, in some cases, deal drugs nonetheless. The drug culture that is so much a part of their lives is one aspect of what Morris Massey* would call their gut level value systems. They are creatures of contemporary values.

Mary is in charge of EMS in the area where Bonnie, Eugene and Albert live and work. Mary, like many of us, has worked hard over the years to develop and maintain a structure of quality assurance for emergency medical services. When federal funds were available, Mary learned that it was important for states, regions and counties to adopt statutes, regulations and ordinances — to make sure that everybody who did EMS was qualified, that they all did EMS as you're supposed to, and that offenders could be penalized by loss of their certification.

In the "old" days, Mary travelled to national EMS conferences sponsored by the federal government. The program was headed by one of the most dynamic and interesting people you would ever want to meet, Dr. David

---

**Morris Massey is a psychologist who developed a theory on how values and beliefs are "programmed" into different age groups. His entertaining, stimulating and ultimately gut-wrenching videotapes explaining his theory have been widely acclaimed, and have enough power to change the way you look at values and behavior. I refer to many of Dr. Massey's ideas thoughout this essay, but I recommend that you view his tapes first-hand. Called "What You Are Is," the tapes can be rented from educational or motivational film distributors. If you can't find a copy, write to us at* JEMS *and we'll locate a distributor.*

Boyd. She listened to Dr. Boyd and others explain their vision of something called "wall-to-wall EMS." Beyond the verbal explanations, there was the federal gospel — Public Law 93-154 and its attendant regulations. As many of us did, Mary found that the message and the gospel was the stuff of a noble and exciting career. She found that it conformed to her gut level values. Then and now, Mary was a creature of traditional values.

Throughout her EMS career, Mary has been selling the message of EMS to others. From about 1972 to about 1982, Mary could relate the message to others in terms of traditional values. I'm sure you've heard some of those terms. "The Congress has determined that serious problems in EMS need to be corrected." "The law requires that prehospital personnel be trained to a minimum level of competence." "The regulations state that you must carry certain equipment on your ambulances." "Failure to comply with the law or the regulations could result in loss of your license or decertification."

Those kinds of statements had predictable impact on most of the people we wanted to change or control. The reactions triggered by those kinds of statements were rooted in the traditional values of respect and obedience for the law, and doing good for the sake of good alone. Those of us who were State EMS Directors at that time found that some of our constituents would fight and argue, to be sure, and some of them would even oppose us at the state legislatures. But, in the end, their traditional values would prevail and they would more or less conform to our regulations and requirements.

About 1982, Mary and others of us began to notice some disturbing changes in attitude. Mostly, the new attitude was exhibited by younger people entering into the field of EMS. They were less compliant. It wasn't that they were defiant or rebellious. It was just that they didn't seem to be moved in any way by the gospel of EMS and the structural guidelines that we had built around it. For a long time, Mary blamed this intangible problem on the loss of federal funding. A lot of us used that as the scapegoat for the changes that were occurring.

I don't know how many of you have read the books of Alvin Toffler, the first one being *Future Shock* (which *was* shocking, and which came true) and the second one, *The Third Wave* (which was equally shocking and which *is* coming true). I don't know how many of you have read John Naisbitt's *Megatrends*. But those authors made big bucks publishing a message that should have been obvious to us. That is, changes that formerly took place on a generational basis (over a period of 25 years or more) now tend to occur in ten years or less. Change has been compacted and accelerated. That should be easy for us to understand. After all, most of us have been the agents of EMS change. Most of us, throughout our careers, have been people who've tried to get others to conform to our way of thinking in this field.

Most of us brought to our roles in EMS the traditional values of the Puritans. As you may recall, the Puritans who founded this country bore a heavy sense of duty to improve both themselves and their community. To the continual irritation and boredom of everybody else, the Puritans were self-righteous. Without feeling the least bit self-conscious, they presumed to have the right and the responsibility to improve other peoples' morals and behavior.

To some extent, that's how most of us undertook the mission of EMS in the 1970's. We were the Puritan circuit riders, carrying the bible of EMS under our arms, and we presumed to improve other peoples' behavior by causing them to conform to our traditional values. We were dissatisfied with the way things had been done, and were being done, and we wanted things done in new and more appropriate ways. In order to meet those goals, we had to confront people with our own EMS values, which, for the most part, were traditional.

Out of that experience, most of us tended to think of ourselves as avant garde. In our minds, most of us had rationalized the limits of individualism versus the needs of society. We were out front in a revolution of emergency medical services. I can remember in the mid-seventies giving a speech by that name — "A Revolution in Health Care." We *were* revolutionaries. We were the symbols of change. We represented the new, the fresh, the forthright, the honest. And many of us still feel that way about ourselves and our roles in this thing called EMS.

Not too long ago, I was in a meeting with Mary (as you'll recall, Mary is an EMS official) and a number of EMS old-timers — those are people who've been involved in EMS for more than five years. At one point, Mary told the audience that her state's process for regulation of EMS was patterned after the federal EMS law and program. As she said it, I looked around the room and a certain attitude of satisfaction could be seen. The gospel of EMS had been formulated by the federal government and the state had fashioned its gospel as a replica of the federal expression of what EMS should be. That made all the folks in the audience — the ones with traditional values — comfortable.

That could be comforting for those of us whose parents were saved from starvation by President Roosevelt's New Deal. For those of us who were raised with the belief that our national government was wise, benevolent and omnipotent, it was comforting to observe that our national government had picked up the banner of EMS, adopted a design for wall-to-wall EMS, and actually spent federal dollars on it. It validated our sense of worth to know that the same national government that created Social Security and won World War II actually believed in this thing called EMS as much as we did. It all fit so neatly into our gut level value systems.

At the same time, as I listened to the veteran EMS official, I found myself wondering about the continuing validity or effectiveness of the federal EMS gospel. How old is it? What was going on in our society when the federal EMS gospel was formulated? What has changed since then?

The federal EMS law which has so influenced our thinking, our processes and our expectations in EMS was first presented to the Congress in 1972. But it reflected the thinking of the period between 1968 and 1972; it was during that time that the concept of regional EMS systems and disease-specific subsystems was born in the minds of some of our pioneers.

What was the American state of mind at the time? The Lyndon Johnson presidency ended and the Nixon presidency began. Viet Nam was omnipresent in our national dialog and conscience. The traditional values of the pre-Watergate era dominated us.

For example, President Johnson's Great Society reflected the belief that the government — through spending and regulation — truly could improve the lives of millions of our less fortunate. As a nation, we tended to believe that anything was possible if we threw enough money at it; we could win any war, we could cure any problem.

That was also the way we approached health care issues in the late sixties and early seventies. We declared war on cancer and threw money at cancer research. The nation was covered with a network of Regional Medical Programs (RMP's), wonderful places to work and play with copious amounts of easy federal dollars. There was some concern about the cost of health care, to be sure, and the Congress created the CHP's, the comprehensive health planning agencies, to deal with that problem. At the same time, hospital construction was rampant and the CAT scanner was introduced. If you think helicopters are a battle now, you should have been around then.

The public generally was unimpressed by efforts to ration health care or contain costs.In those times, it was unfashionable to mention money and lifesaving in the same breath. There were no limits to what we would do or what we would spend to save a life. In those early days of selling EMS to reluctant county commissioners or state legislators, how many of us said, "Yes, it is expensive, but if it saves just one life it'll be worth it"?

On the fringes of all this were some noisy and irritating people who challenged our federal government's military adventures. For the most part, this was the same noisy and irritating group of people who upset the tranquility of college campuses with profanity, dirty clothes, long hair, and political militancy. It seemed to most of us that Mayor Daley's method of dealing with these people was the ultimate solution. Our traditional values told us that there should be regulations to control such outrageous behavior and those regulations should be sternly enforced.

Some of us had small children during those years when the modern view of EMS was coalescing and being put on paper as policy. Those children are the second generation of Americans to spend their entire lives under the threat of nuclear annihilation. They are the first full generation of Americans to spend their entire lives watching the world, including a war, on color television.

Those people who were children during the formation of modern EMS policy would become the first generation of Americans to be exposed to illegal drugs in their elementary schoolyards. They would become the first generation of Americans to see their nation lose a war, and to see a President resign in disgrace. Before reaching adulthood, they would learn that people on the other side of the world could radically alter our lifestyle and its cost by simply shutting off an oil valve. They are the generation of Americans who would plead with their parents on Saturday night to stay up late — so they could watch "Emergency!" on TV.

That was the environment in which our EMS gospel was born. For many of us, it was an atmosphere of boundless ideals and ambitions. Prior to 1973, we believed our nation to be capable of anything, regardless of cost. We had been conditioned to carry the heavy burden of the Puritans and the notion that we had some personal responsibility for the well being of society. Those traditional values made it OK for us to presume that we could change and improve other people's behavior if necessary to match our vision of a better society.

But how do you change or influence the performance and behavior of others? In one way or another, that's what every one of us is all about — getting people to do things, and do those things the way we want them done. People like Eugene and Bonnie and Albert. People who Morris Massey would say may be different than us but who are, nonetheless, one hundred percent normal. Typical people with contemporary values. People whose values were formed since the assassination of John F. Kennedy.

By virtue of our positions, just about all of us will have temporary opportunities to control the behavior and performance of other people. Think about that.

Throughout human history, the right to control other people has been the rallying point for revolution, conquest and war between nations. Somewhere deep in our genetic make-up, most of us have an impulse to try to control the behavior and performance of other people. In an earlier time, when the people we worked with or supervised shared our traditional values, controlling their behavior was mostly a matter of establishing rules and enforcing them if necessary. Usually, enforcement was not necessary. People with traditional values respect and need secure employment.

But for most people with contemporary values, their current position is "just a job" that they'll stick with until something better comes along. Morris Massey tells about the situation where an employer issuing discipline tells his employee, "You get two days off without pay!" The employee bounces back with the question, "Can I have five?"

Those of you who have traditional values know that you are able to provide much of your own positive reinforcement. By contrast, people with contemporary values need frequent positive reinforcement from management. Those of you who have traditional values tend to trust your boss until severely disappointed. The person with contemporary values, by contrast, tends to suspect or distrust management until management proves it can be trusted.

The EMS gospel in the U.S., that revered foundation upon which we have built our careers and our expectations, was dependent on traditional values. It was semi-military; it dealt with national standards, uniform specifications, guidelines and regulations, governing bodies, rules, responsibilities and non-negotiable conditions for funding. The penalties for non-compliance ranged from defunding to decertification.

In the early 1970's, that's about all it took to make a program work — or, at least, seem to work. The tools of enforcement included fear — fear of losing a job, fear of diminished chances for promotion, fear of decertification, fear of being held in contempt or ridicule by one's peers, fear of not conforming to the norm.

Those things don't work anymore. When people see their job as a place to be until something better comes along, you can't alter or control their behavior by threatening to take their job away. Remember, the people whose behavior you are trying to alter or control are the very same people who spent their most impressionable years seeing the threat of nuclear war on TV, witnessing their country lose a war, making ethical choices about drugs and sex while still in elementary school.

If you expect these people to be impressed by threats to take away their certification or their jobs, forget it. You are dealing with a generation which has seen a President chased from office while corporate executives ravaged the environment without penalty. You are dealing with a generation that has seen elected officials at every level charged or convicted of theft or dishonesty. They have seen the poor crooks go to jail while the rich and privileged crooks did not. Every day, they and their fellow citizens violate a national 55 mph speed limit — and get away with it.

So things are different than they once were. Things will always be different than they once were. We've all heard old-timers grumble about how things aren't the way they used to be. We've all had a boss who's grumbled about how the world is going to hell. Maybe so, but in the meantime, we've got a responsibility to control the performance and behavior of others. How do we do that?

Ray Kroc, the founder of McDonald's, had a system. He and his people created a 700-page book of regulations on how to fry and serve a hamburger. For a long time, you could stop at the Golden Arches in Revere, Massachusetts, Fort Dodge, Iowa, or Medford, Oregon, and buy the identical product, served exactly the same. Ray Kroc had traditional values and his company has delivered those values to millions of people billions of times.

If it worked for Ray Kroc, why can't it work for us? Why can't we write a 700-page book on how to deliver emergency medical services? Why can't we impose traditional values on the system as McDonald's has on hamburgers?

In my judgment, there are several reasons why the cookbook approach to controlling the performance and behavior of others will not work in EMS. In the first place, providing emergency medical services (especially in a prehospital setting) is far more complex than cooking and selling hamburgers. Secondly, the people of our organizations generally are of a different composition than minimum wage frycooks and teenage counter attendants. Thirdly, who says it's good to have total uniformity? Finally, there are signs that it's not even working for McDonald's anymore.

Probably my biggest gripe with the cookbook approach to hamburgers or EMS is the matter of uniformity. All of us, at one time or another, without realizing we were doing it, have exhibited a psycho-social flaw. We have made it obvious that we would feel much more comfortable if things were all alike, if they looked the same, if they functioned the same, if they didn't surprise or confound us with irritating distinctions or differences.

One of my dearest friends in all the world is Leo Schwartz, the retired chief of the EMS bureau at NHTSA.

Leo spent nearly 50 years working for government, and it affected certain aspects of his thinking and his personality. For example, he had a fetish about the color of ambulances. He wanted all ambulances in the U.S. to be white with a 14" wide band of contrasting Omaha Orange paint.

The fact is, uniformity is the seedbed of self-satisfied isolationism and mediocrity. Everybody who has ever made an exceptional contribution to our society has broken from the constraints of mediocrity to do so — even Leo Schwartz. Uniformity usually is promoted in the form of minimum standards. But "minimum standards" is just another way of defining the worst that we will let things get before we have to do something about it.

I realize these are fighting words to people who have spent years of their lives in the process of developing and adopting minimum standards for EMS. I realize the discomfort you may feel about my suggestions that uniformity is bad. I suspect that some of you, within the last few minutes, have briefly considered your perception of the alternative — a grab bag of different people, all doing their own thing as their individual value systems command them to. What kind of a system would that be? Is that what I'm suggesting as an alternative to uniformity? No! So long as the public expects us to do for them what they are unable to do for themselves, it will be necessary for us to be predictable and reliable — and that requires some degree of uniformity. The difference is how we arrive at what must be uniform and to what extent. The difference is the process by which we set standards and enforce them — or, even better, arrange for them to enforce themselves.

Eugene and Bonnie and Albert are very typical — and if you don't believe that, you are not in touch with your world. Eugene and Bonnie and Albert are living proof that we no longer have the easy advantage of unquestioned compliance with authority. No longer can we count on a rulebook to serve as our sword and our shield. The way we do things in the future will be hammered out through an ongoing consensus process.

As it becomes obvious that rules and regulations no longer command the respect of the governed or meet the needs of those served, they will be replaced by value statements. Those value statements will be generated by a process involving everybody in the system. Traditional and contemporary values will collide in the process; turmoil and conflict over the content of value statements will preoccupy the entire system. Those who enter the process with contemporary values will emerge with more traditional values.

There may be some surprising outcomes. For example, I've been experimenting with the process — using some young people who are very much representative of contemporary values. I have given them an opportunity to establish their own expectations — to set standards against which they consent to be judged. We call them value statements, and we arrive at them through a consensus process.

Much to my surprise, these young people, when given an opportunity to formally define standards for their own performance, usually are tougher on themselves than I would have been. Furthermore, they have a pride of authorship, a psychic ego investment in their value statements, and a defensiveness for those self-imposed standards that results in self-policing within their peer group.

What a refreshing alternative to rebellion against unseen authorities who impose rules, regulations, protocols, policies and procedures from on high. Creating and maintaining value statements (as an alternative to traditional regulation) is a process. In the old days, when we undertook some kind of process, we would conclude that the published result was an end point. For example, we would issue a memo, or a training bulletin, or amend the rules and regulations. "OK, that's done. On to the next problem." In the case of building value statements by consensus, there is no end point. The process is ongoing. Every value statement is forever temporary, always anticipating the impact of megatrends, economics, changed public needs, and the infusion of newer and younger people (bringing with them — God forbid — still different values).

Within about ten years you're going to be faced with a whole new group of people to be supervised who bring to their jobs values that are completely foreign to those that you now have. You — the generation who are just breaking out of contemporary values and trying your best to conform to traditional values — are going to find that you will be faced with this problem in less than a decade. And then *they* will, but maybe it won't take ten years. Maybe it'll take just five, six or seven before the next wave of people (raised in the information age, raised with computers in their bedrooms) will be confronting you. Who knows? Maybe, they'll be more traditional than their predecessors. The point is we've got to be flexible, and the systems we use to control and influence the behavior of other people this year may not work next year.

For those who fear change, for those who cannot tolerate people and ideas different than their own, these are bad times — and they will get worse. For those who need to control the behavior of others through dogma and mandates, I can offer no comfort. Those who rely on rules and regulations to achieve uniformity will need to prepare quickly for a wiggly world where virtually everybody possesses the power to veto the rules and regulations. Those who coast from crisis to crisis, executing quick fixes in between, face a distressing future where solutions are never complete and the process for reaching them is never finished.

If you're inclined not to believe all this, if you consider this message radical nonsense, just remember that Eugene and Bonnie and Albert and others like them work in my system and they work in your system. Remember that the essence of our jobs is to influence or control the behavior or performance of others. Remember that those "others" increasingly are different than you and me, but that doesn't make them bad. As Massey says, they are a hundred percent normal. We have to remember that their gut level value systems were formed around a completely different set of influences and stimuli.

For example, one of the things that Massey talked about was music. Now, my kids would probably say that I'm almost "with it." The young people whom I supervise might think of me as a "progressive" boss. But they can't imagine a time when the most popular song in America was called, "How much is that doggy in the window?" That happened when I was in high school, when my values were being formed. And if I tell them that, with the heavy metal sounds of Iron Maiden playing in the background, do you think they'd consider me weird? You're damned right they would.

Given those differences, we've got to remember that the bottom line in our conventional systems of control is the threat of decertification, loss of job, or misdemeanor penalties. And we've got to remember that people like Bonnie the nurse, Eugene the EMT, and Albert the emergency physician are willing to face those risks every Saturday night. They thumb their noses at the "authority." How can we expect them to be impressed with our regulations?

I don't know what's going on in your heads as you consider this message and its implications. Maybe you're frightened. Maybe you're mad. But I am enthusiastic — excited — grateful for an opportunity to be in a position of influence in some of the most dynamic times in the history of mankind.

I'm thankful that I stumbled across this concept, the Massey tapes, the opportunity to supervise young people, a few accidents of history involving my children and other young adults, that have really jolted me.I'm thankful for that. Because wouldn't it be awful to go down that old road of traditional values, increasingly bitter with the changes in life, not understanding them, constantly being threatened by them, gradually retreating into a safe little cocoon of traditional behavior and rejection of anything else, to the point where we stood alone, withering and dying and waiting for the grim reaper to come and sweep us away? Instead, we have an opportunity to recognize these wonderful changes, this quick succession of events that is shaping the world and each generation as it comes along, and be a part of it. It may, indeed, be one of the real opportunities to defy the natural inclination that starts the day we are born — namely, decay.

Possibly for the first time in history of EMS, human resources have found their way to the front burner. If we are to be successful, serious attention to the people of EMS is a must. Never again will people take a back seat to transfer agreements, trauma center designations, grant applications, radio repeaters, and the paint schemes of ambulances.

As the next few years come and go in our field, one of the most common words in our vocabulary will become obsolete. That word is "management." In this new age, managers will fail while leaders excel. People will refuse to be managed, but they will hunger for competent leadership.

As traditional values clash with contemporary values, our field will need an abundant supply of humanistic leaders. It will be necessary for those leaders to launch career-length processes of participative governance, including development of organizational values through consensus. It's hard, and it takes time, and it upsets work habits developed over the prior years.

We are going to need to reject uniformity for the sake of uniformity, and reject form when it stands in the way of function. Most of all, we will need to recognize instinctively the human elements that distinguish emergency medical services from hamburgers.

Let's face it. None of us are getting any younger. Most of us have chosen to work in influential roles in the exciting field of EMS. A major part of that job involves the effort to control and influence the behavior and performance of other people. The people we now need to control and influence have a different set of "hot" buttons than those who worked in EMS ten years ago. If we continue to try to control and influence behavior and performance with methods that are outdated and no longer work, we are wasting much of the diminishing amount of time we have left. As we have observed in others, there's nothing quite so sad as one who finishes a career out of touch, out of power, and not understanding what went wrong.

5

People and Places

One of the Boys

It was May 11, 1971, when my path first crossed that of Robert A. Cinader. We met at Fire Station 7 in West Hollywood. He offered me a job, researching potential story material for a proposed television series. It was a turning point in my life, with both good and bad consequences.

Bob Cinader presented himself in a kind of stoop-shouldered indifference to physical appearances. More often than not, his facial expressions were a mix of frowns and scowls. In meeting or greeting him, one could expect a report on numerous ills, pains and inconveniences,

I never knew very much about his childhood or adolescence in New York. I presume he was a kid who couldn't master stickball but made up for it with his mastery of the written word. Bob Cinader was brilliant, one of the greatest minds I have ever encountered.

Bob died of cancer in November, 1982. Probably, in his final days, he thought about his life, its high points and lows. Certainly, his long marriage to a lovely lady must have ranked high in his life achievements. But I would guess that the summer of '71 also would be classed as one of his fondest memories. It was then that Bob Cinader (possibly for the first time) became "one of the boys."

Our early research had resulted in selling the concept of "Emergency!" to NBC. Bob's task was to develop a script for a world premiere TV movie, although producer Jack Webb would get most of the credit for it. Already, there was talk of a weekly series spinning off from the world premiere. Bob Cinader would be executive producer of the one-hour shows and he had just a few weeks to get acquainted with the world of firefighters and paramedics.

By that time, I was a battalion chief in a 60 sq. mi. region of South L.A. For several weeks, Bob Cinader accompanied me on my tours of duty. At first, in deference to a film producer in their midst, the firefighters and paramedics were still and polite. But after a few days they reverted to form. I remember the first time Cinader got "stuck in the tank" (forced to wash dishes) after losing a hand of firehouse poker. He complained, and scowled, but I think he loved being treated as one of the boys.

As we traveled throughout Battalion 7, visiting fire stations and hospitals, rolling on fires and emergency calls, he became less an attraction. The "real" people would greet him with a "Hi, Bob." In the back seat of my red sedan, he would talk endlessly between puffs on his foul smelling cigarillo. My driver and I heard more than we ever wanted to know about the Los Angeles Police Department and "Adam 12" (which he had produced). But as the days passed his devotion to paramedics and EMS became a passion which would have no rival in his remaining years.

As we all know, Bob Cinader's "Emergency!" series

became a huge success. More than 120 one-hour segments were produced over a six-year period. Some segments have been re-run as many as nine times in the U.S.

Bob Cinader's passion for EMS and the fire service got him appointed to L.A. County's Paramedic Commission. He tended to immerse himself in the turbulent politics of L.A. County's EMS system. His strong opinions and his dominating style produced for him as many enemies as friends. There were those who suggested that he was ill-prepared to design or govern a health care system.

Prepared or not, there have been few people who have had more influence on any aspect of health care. In his docu-drama approach to presenting "Emergency!", Bob Cinader elevated America's (indeed, the world's) expectations. No new concept in health care has spread as rapidly as prehospital ALS (paramedic) services. One main reason is the public education which was accomplished through an unusual prime-time TV series.

He may never have been good at stickball. But his mind, his talents, and his dogged persistence produced a message that profoundly affected people throughout North America. Without Bob Cinader's TV show, paramedics might have become a brief experiment in a few cities. Instead, countless lives have been saved.

I wish I had known he was dying. I would have tried to let him know the importance of his contribution. In the process, I would have let him know that I liked him best with suds up to his elbows — stuck in the tank as one of the boys.

Don't You Hate Zealots?

Don't you just hate people who try to convert you to their way of life? Like the guy who traded alcoholism for fundamentalist religion and then hounds you to become just like him. Or the Amway saleslady who's convinced that signing you up will make you as happy and fulfilled as the folks in their TV commercial.

Several months ago, in Des Moines, I found myself in the midst of some physical fitness zealots. I could have escaped, but a beautiful lady had struck up a conversation with me and, well. . . . I was enjoying it. Her golden hair flowed gracefully over her shoulders. Her skin was smooth and taut and bronze.

I was trying to be attentive to the conversation. "It's not a matter of living forever," she was saying. "Being physically fit makes our lives so much more enjoyable." Her eyes sparkled with enthusiasm and I struggled to pay attention to what she was saying.

When I regained control of my concentration, she was

talking about smoking. "I just don't understand how people can destroy their health with that disgusting habit," she said. "Most of the nurses I work with (she's a nurse!) see the results of smoking every day, and they still smoke. How can anyone take care of COPD patient, or an emphysema patient, or a lung cancer patient, and still go on smoking?"

After an awkward moment, I realized she was expecting an answer from me. "I don't smoke," I blurted clumsily. Another awkward moment slowly passed. My mind raced for a change of subject. "By the way, if you're a nurse, you may have seen a magazine called *JEMS*," I offered hopefully. After we had established that an EMT friend of hers keeps the current *JEMS* on his coffee table (to impress the girls?) and that I was the publisher of said journal, she launched back into her favorite topic.

"You should have a regular column in the magazine — about physical fitness," she continued. "I'm single (she's single!) and I've dated some of the EMTs. Most of them would really be attractive if they would just get in shape. They're carrying too much weight, they don't get any meaningful aerobic exercise, and they're going to look much older than their years if they don't get fit. About a year ago, I decided I wouldn't date guys who smoke."

"I don't smoke," I blurted clumsily.

"Why doesn't your magazine sponsor some mini-marathons or fun runs around the country?" the pretty lady asked with widened eyes and a broad smile which revealed beautiful white teeth. While I groped for an answer, she continued to evangelize. "There's *no* way people can stay healthy unless they eat right and get plenty of daily aerobic exercise. You've got to do *both*. I set aside an hour every day just for me. Whether it's running, or aerobic dancing, or riding my bicycle, I follow the 'TPB 30' principle."

My mind raced, trying to figure out what 'TPB 30' was all about. Finally, concluding there was no other way to respond, I asked, "What is that. . . TPB 30?"

She knew I was stumped. She knew I could never walk away from that angelic smile and the attentive gaze of those gorgeous eyes. "It stands for temperature, pulse and breathing. The "30" refers to 30 minutes. In order to get in good shape and stay there, you must elevate your body temperature, your pulse and your breathing — all at the same time — and keep them elevated for at least 30 minutes every day."

"You certainly are a walking advertisement for physical fitness," I said. She smiled, placed her hands on her hips, thrust out her bosom, and turned in a slow pirouette. "Thanks," she said, "but you should have seen me three years ago," "You?" I replied with exaggerated surprise. "Yep, a real widebody. . . and a smoker too."

The conversation concluded when the lady's boyfriend hailed her from across the room. She bid me a friendly good-bye and bounced off with her skinny friend.

As I said, don't you just hate people who try to convert you to their way of life? It seems that every physical fitness evangelist is intent on getting the rest of the world in shape. The biggest obstacle is holding your attention long enough to get the message across. I hope I have succeeded.

The Hands-Down Expert

On a summer morning in 1966, I pulled my sagging VW into the parking lot of fire station 69 in Topanga Canyon. I was a new fire captain and this was to be my assignment — 42 miles from home. A red Plymouth sedan was parked in front of the station. That could only mean one thing.

As I walked into the station with my arms filled with turnout gear, Harvey Anderson sized me up sternly and grunted a reluctant "good morning." He was the division chief and supreme commander of the several hundred square miles of mountains, canyons, flammable brush and timber that circles the north and west of the Los Angeles basin. I had never worked for Harvey before but I'd heard about him (". . . a tyrant — eats captains alive").

Harvey is a self-made man. He grew up in the worst of the Depression and worked his way through the University of California. When he joined the fire department's forestry division, he was distinctive from the first day. The foresters did a lot of pick and shovel work in those days and Harvey Anderson, with his college degree, could work circles around any of his brawny counterparts.

Many of the fire breaks in the mountains around L.A. were first cut by hand. Harvey was among those who cut them. They used horses and mules to get to and from their work projects. Harvey usually hiked, pulling the mules behind him. As time passed, he came to know every nook and cranny of his future brush fire battlefields.

He rose through the ranks till he got to his level of peak competence. Long before Dr. Lawrence Peter wrote about his "Peter Principle," Harvey Anderson stopped seeking promotions which would remove him from what he did best: manage major emergencies. I've seen Harvey Anderson covered with the grime of a campaign brush fire, standing at the peak of a mountain with radio in hand, surveying his battlefield and commanding a dazzling array of resources as few men could.

He was good at it for several reasons. He knew the terrain — he had hiked every mile of it. He knew the enemy — he knew the botanical pedigree, the calorific fuel value, and the combustion characteristics of the Southern California watershed vegetation. He had experience — he had fought fires on the same ground every few years and he remembered those battles. He knew how to use his resources — he used aircraft for strategy, not TV cameras. He used tractors, hand labor crews, and pumpers for greatest effect and least hazard to life. Most important, he knew his people — he would assign a big sector of a fire to a young captain whom he trusted while telling an office chief to "get the hell outta my way."

In 1968, Harvey Anderson became the victim of a dumb law. He was forced to retire simply because he turned 60 years old. He came to my station in the final hours of his last day on the job. True to his nature, he didn't wind down into retirement. He was on the phone, taking care of business, until the clock forced him to stop.

Since 1968, Harvey has been busy saving lives. For as long as I've known him, he's been running five miles every day. He's become a physical fitness consultant and he'll tell you more than you ever wanted to know about the subject. He's transferred much of his uncommon energy and zeal to the subject of preventive health and particularly blood pressure screening and management. For several years, he's served as chairman of the Physical Fitness Committee of the International Association of Fire Chiefs. In recent years, he's been traveling to the Grand Canyon to teach physical fitness to forest rangers.

My first encounter with Harvey Anderson was not a meeting. It was a collision of personalities. He won and I benefited. As we witness the clay-footed performance of so many supervisors and administrators in today's world of public service, I only wish that more people could have shared my opportunity to see a real boss do his job as nobody else could. When you know your boss is the hands-down expert and has the courage to stand for what's right, it's hard not to be loyal.

POSTSCRIPT: As this book was going to press, we heard from Harvey Anderson. He was alive and well — on the beach at Malibu. At age 78, he walks six miles a day and continues to promote physical fitness ("It's one-hundred percent certain that we're all gonna die, so why not die healthy?," he asks).

A Message from the Coroner

In 1972, the Los Angeles County paramedic program was on the brink of termination. The financial support to continue and expand the program just wasn't there. Then, quite suddenly, the County Board of Supervisors found more than $600,000 to continue and expand the program. With one magnanimous gesture, control of the fledgling program was grabbed from doctors and handed to politicians and bureaucrats. Since that magic moment, things have been going downhill.

There have been opportunities for the doctors to regain control in the interim. Apparently, it hasn't occurred to them. Meanwhile, so-called "base station hospitals" have spread like ameobae, bad habits have proliferated throughout the (non) system, some patients have been hurt, some lawsuits have popped up, and everybody seems to wait for the next crisis or accident to grab the stage and

NOTE: This appeared in the August, 1980 issue of JEMS.

put forth his own pet opinions on what's wrong.

One recent example involved a 42-year-old man who was seen by paramedics in an apparent state of unconsciousness. After testing the patient's responses they concluded that the man was feigning his comatose state. They left the scene without making a consultation with their base hospital and the man died in bed a few hours later of a "massive brain hemorrhage."

Later, the paramedics found themselves at the center of a public controversy. They were called to testify at a coroner's inquest and the story commanded three columns in the *Los Angeles Times*. The coroner's jury ruled that the death was accidental but made some recommendations "to improve emergency care by paramedics."

The first recommendation was that legislation be enacted to establish statewide paramedic standards. That's not a bad idea but, since L.A. County is acknowledged as having one of the highest paramedic training standards in California, it's hard to see how legislation would have made a difference in this case.

The second recommendation: "That paramedics always function under, and be in radio contact with, their base station physicians." Oh, yeah? What if they have several to choose from (the "dial-a-doc" syndrome)? What if the personnel at those "base station" hospitals don't fully understand their responsibility to or relationship with those voices at the other end of the radio? Radio contact without some formal ongoing relationship between paramedic and emergency physician (trainer-trainee, supervisor-subordinate, auditor-performer, master-servant) will be just that — radio contact.

The third recommendation calls for thorough logs (records) to be maintained on all cases. We welcome Los Angeles County to the rest of the world. Also, we urge somebody at the Hall of Administration to check the overflowing "in" baskets. A proposal for a complete EMS data system has been sitting there since 1973.

The fourth and final recommendation is that paramedics stress to families of victims the need to contact their own physicians on all calls. Oh, brother! That's all we need.

The modern concept of prehospital advanced life support is based on the following structure: Fully qualified and fully authorized emergency physicians in a limited number of qualified and specially designated hospitals utilize the trained employees of another agency or organization ("borrowed servants") to deliver advanced life support services as an outreach function of the hospital. To the extent that individuals avail themselves of this system of emergency care, they must accept the fact that it is a public system designed to serve the greatest possible number of patients with efficiency and safety, to the extent of available resources. The necessary efficiency and safety can be achieved only through a formal relationship between the authorized emergency physician and the paramedic surrogates operating under his command. The integrity of the system requires that other physicians intervene in the care of patients only with the express permission of the authorized emergency physician.

Emergency physicians in L.A. need to come in out of the sun and recapture their emergency care system. It's just not fair to expect paramedics to work in a system that has no medical control. There should be a message in the fact that a *coroner's jury* has tried to alter the operation of the (non)system. The politicians have had control for eight years. The results have been deadly.

POSTSCRIPT: Since 1980, the legislation to establish statewide (minimum) standards has been enacted and the state and local EMS bureaucracies have produced volumes of regulations. Still, local certification prevails and county lines are barriers to paramedics and their employers.

The proliferation of so-called "base station hospitals" in L.A. has been controlled but the bigness of the system still is offered by many as an excuse for design defects. Through it all, the health bureaucracy has been staffed by true believers who give heart and soul to the system. Currently, they are developing a county-wide data collection system — 16 years overdue but welcome nonetheless.

Despite our challenge for emergency physicians to recapture the EMS system in L.A., it still remains the property of politicians. All in all, Los Angeles' is the best of the nation's really big EMS systems — but it could have been so much better.

The Call Didn't Come

Bob Schreiber was a paramedic in New York City. Like most of his colleagues in the Big Apple's creaky EMS system, he lived with the day-to-day frustrations of "backlogs" and delayed responses. Too often, he and his partner had to answer to angry citizens for problems they had no control over. How do you convince a new widow in Staten Island that the 50-minute delay was the fault of some anonymous dispatcher in Queens?

In the final minutes of his life, Bob Schreiber became the victim of two life-threatening crises. One, an apparent heart attack, robbed him of his life while the other, apparent human incompetence, deprived him of any chance for survival. The system he had served for six years failed him in his time of greatest need.

Schreiber was at his Staten Island home when stricken. His wife, certified in CPR, called 911 for help, and then

---

NOTE: This appeared in the May, 1980 issue of JEMS.

started CPR on her husband. The call was logged with the police and with the EMS dispatch center in Queens at 11:52 p.m. The nearest city paramedic unit was available in its quarters and waiting for a call. The call didn't come.

New York's police dispatchers have come to expect mysterious foul-ups at the EMS dispatch center and they've learned to work around the system. At 12:15 a.m., twenty-three minutes after they had called the EMS dispatchers, the cops called a Staten Island volunteer rescue squad. The volunteers arrived at Schreiber's home five minutes later but they could not perform advanced life support procedures. The Staten Island paramedic unit still had not been notified by their dispatcher; they finally received the alarm at 12:31 a.m. — 39 minutes after Mrs. Schreiber had placed her call. It was an 11-minute response and when they arrived — *fifty minutes after the original call* — it was too late.

Next day, the operations director of New York City EMS suspended an unidentified dispatcher and launched an investigation. A few days after Bob Schreiber's funeral, I traveled to New York City and was treated to both sides of the delay story.

First, there was a tour of the dispatch center. It's a very busy place. It includes one of the first and most successful call screening operations in the county. The little cards that slide along a conveyor belt begin to look like little cards after a few minutes. You have to remind yourself that each of them represents a human being, some of whom are dying at that very moment.

My tour of the establishment was conducted by a long-time friend, a man who literally vibrates with his commitment to high quality and efficient EMS. But he doesn't hold all the reins; he is only one of several who direct and control EMS in America's biggest city. Dutifully, he impressed me with his knowledge of the system, the sheer volume of it all, and some exciting plans for future improvements. At the same time, he looked worried.

I spent the rest of the day with New York City paramedics. Like astronauts and fighter pilots, they have the "right stuff." They are well trained. They are totally committed to their profession. They are tough but still sensitive. And they are fighting mad!

The paramedics claimed the logjam was in the EMS dispatch center. They place the blame on the people who staff that place. And they blame the system's administrators for trying to deny, hide or pacify the problem. The City's EMS bosses had labeled the paramedics "rabble-rousers." But my instincts told me the paramedics were right.

Then I heard from a legislative investigator. He told me the dispatcher on Bob Schreiber's case had been on the job for only 80 days, but that he had been absent from work for 68 of those days. Reportedly, this person had severe problems with diction and possibly suffered from dyslexia. While Bob Schreiber was waiting for an ambulance, the dispatcher was busy getting names and numbers for a shift change report.

"Rabble-rousers," indeed. Hasn't anybody noticed that the paramedics simply are pushing for the opportunity to do their job as they were trained? These are bright young people who want to serve to the best of their ability, and there is an unaccountable obstacle in their way. People of lesser constitution might become as silent and mechanistic as those little cards that slide along the conveyor.

POSTSCRIPT: Writing this piece, I faced for the first time the dilemma of a story versus a friendship. The story needed to be told,

I felt. Never before had an EMS publication investigated and reported a local problem with real candor. I wanted to establish the price to be paid for letting an EMS system get sloppy. I felt that our field could never mature so long as serious and deadly problems were being denied by administrators and ignored by publishers. This column had an impact on New York City, and it set a new standard for EMS journalism. It hurt a friend who thought I had come to praise him, but it fortified some good paramedics who were much more than just "rabble-rousers."

Since 1980, major strides have been made by New York City EMS in reducing response times. But the system has developed a pattern of peaks and valleys — and we've reported both. In October '85, for example, we commented on an effort by one of the mayor's key aides to restructure medical control of the EMS system. Since then, the aide was forced to admit that his educational credentials were phony and he resigned in disgrace.

Twenty Years Later

Most everybody who was more than 10 years old when President Kennedy was assassinated can tell you where he was and what he was doing when the awful news reached him. But how many can remember where they were and what they were doing when the National Academy of Science-National Research Council (NAS-NRC) published their report, "Accidental Death and Disability: The Neglected Disease of Modern Society?"

My memories of that year are vivid. I was a young fire captain in 1966, based at the Topanga Canyon fire station between Malibu and the San Fernando Valley. Our first-in district included many miles of winding mountain roads. We were the only full-time public agency located in a

---

NOTE: This appeared in the May, 1986 issue of JEMS *as part of a commentary on the twentieth anniversary of the report, "Accidental Death and Disability: The Neglected Disease of Modern Society."*

75-square-mile area. We were first on-scene at every vehicle accident — and there were lots of them. A typical wait for an ambulance was 20 minutes to an hour.

At the time, we thought we were quite good at rescue and first aid. On the other hand, nobody had taught us the importance of immobilizing necks. We didn't know how to apply traction to fractured femurs. Our suction equipment consisted of a gas-powered aspirator on our E&J Lytport resuscitator (which did not include a demand valve at that time).

There were no EMS magazines or newsletters available in 1966. We could not start IVs, intubate airways, or administer drugs. We had no backboards. The stokes stretcher was our basic tool for moving patients. I remember my crew devising some eleborate winch arrangements for getting injured people up out of steep canyons. I remember receiving a new Advanced First Aid card in the mail (with my name on it) even though I had not received any refresher training or taken a recertification test.

When the ambulance (an International Carry-All) arrived, we would help the attendants load the patients. In our minds, that was the end of the case. Where the patients were going or how they would be cared for didn't occur to us. At the time, our experience and our training did not incline us to think of rescue and first-aid work as part of a system. We did our job, the ambulance guys did theirs, and we presumed the hospital people did theirs. In our minds, the only real flaw in the system was the long response times for the ambulance.

Three or four more years would pass before I became fully aware of the NAS-NRC "White Paper." By that time, my career and my life had been altered by some important efforts to improve prehospital emergency medical care. But those efforts were completely independent of the NAS-NRC report. They were the products of cardiologists, not surgeons. They occurred largely as a result of informal communications between a handful of doctors, rather than the effort of any national group or organization.

Though significance of the so-called White Paper should not be diminished in any way, it would be unjust to overlook the contributions of cardiology to what we now know as modern EMS.

One of the most important EMS pioneers in the free world was J. Frank Pantridge, MD. In 1963, he was physician in charge of the Department of Cardiology at the Royal Victoria Hospital in Belfast, Northern Ireland. Concerned with the out-of-hospital death rate for myocardial infarction, he established a system for getting advanced life support *to* the patient in the field, before the patient arrived at the hospital. To accomplish this task, he employed *non*-physicians to deliver mobile coronary care.

Let's face it. In 1966, the surgeons who influenced the White Paper were thinking about sending doctors into the field to rendezvous with ambulances properly equipped to meet *their* needs. Pantridge, by comparison, had already proven that trained technicians (non-physicians) could make dramatic differences in the outcome of life-threatening medical emergencies if they reached the patient soon enough in the field.

Pantridge's work didn't get published until 1967.[†] Earlier, however, he had traveled to the U.S. and spoken of his program at cardiology conferences. As the NAS-NRC White Paper was being published, several cardiologists already were following Pantridge's lead and designing prehospital programs that would greatly benefit emergency cardiac patients and also trauma victims. In fact, early in

1967, Dr. Eugene Nagel (an anesthesiologist who traveled to cardiology meetings) authorized our nation's first paramedics to function on the streets of Miami.

The White Paper inspired important developments, to be sure, including development of a national curriculum for "Emergency Medical Technician" (a new title, intended to replace "ambulance attendant"). But, in several localities, the cardiologists were training and fielding paramedics (Columbus, Seattle, Los Angeles) to provide prehospital advanced life support before EMT training programs were even available.

By that time, I was a fire captain in West Hollywood and received a visit from a television producer. He wanted to produce a TV series about "rescue" (whatever that was) but wasn't interested in paramedics. ("America's not ready for a heart attack every Saturday night," he once said.) I put him in the hands of some cardiologists and some paramedics and the rest is history.

Again, I don't mean to diminish the contribution of the watershed document of our field, or the people who wrote it. On the other hand, it is clear that the White Paper was only one of several significant events which would mold the future of prehospital emergency care. Probably, without the rapid-fire development of mobile coronary care units and the subsequent impact of a primetime TV show, the average citizen still would be thinking of trauma as a mental disease.

Twenty years later, some highly vocal and visible surgeons are pressing for a return to "scoop and run" basic ambulance service for trauma patients. Of course, few of them have spent any significant time riding as an observer on busy ambulance units. Twenty years later, more than half of all U.S. residents are within a few minutes of an advanced life support paramedic unit, and they aren't about to give up their paramedics — no matter what the academic surgeons say.

Twenty years later, the Emergency Cardiac Care Committee of the American Heart Association continues to dominate standard-setting for prehospital advanced life support. The White Paper called for the establishment of a national trauma association; the American Trauma Society was the result but it's always been a store without merchandise, managed by people who are very good at something else.

At *JEMS*, we occupy a unique vantage point for judging the current status of EMS. The letters, article submissions, photographs and news clippings we receive tell us a lot about how far EMS has come since publication of the NAS-NRC report in 1966. Some of it reminds me of my tenure as a fire captain in Topanga Canyon 20 years ago.

We still see evidence of rescue and ambulance personnel who don't bother to immobilize potentially unstable necks. We see pictures of patients being moved without backboard (in 1986!). We hear about ambulance personnel (including certified EMTs) who know little if anything about suction and suction equipment. We've witnessed cases where EMTs have been certified or recertified without demonstrating their competence to perform basic life support.

What has been accomplished during this 20-year period? In some places, a complete turnaround in prehospital and in-hospital emergency care. In other places, a short period of effort to improve, followed by a longer period of benign neglect and apathy. Even worse, there are places in the U.S. where ill or injured people receive the same kind of field treatment and transportation they received in 1966 or earlier.

In re-reading the White Paper after all these years, I

noted that the recommendations, for the most part, were structural. Form committees, implement legislation, delineate radio frequencies, develop trauma registries, autopsy victims, conduct research in trauma. It was the Lyndon Johnson era and all except the "hippies" were impressed by the structural approach to making change.

A colleague, Jimm Murray, chief of Wyoming's EMS office, has alluded to changed attitudes and lesser commitments on the part of many field EMS personnel providers. We know what he's talking about and it bothers us a lot. If there were a new opportunity to write another White Paper on EMS, we would insist that it include lots of thought and words on how to motivate everybody in the system — from EMT to trauma surgeon. In my view, the neglected disease of 1986 is the shortage or absence of true compassion among care givers. Even with all the structural pieces anticipated by the 1966 report, the machine of EMS will work correctly only if it is fueled by the unquenchable desire to do good for the sake of good alone.

---

†*Pantridge, J.F., and Geddes, J.S. "A Mobile Intensive Care Unit in the Management of Myocardial Infarction."* Lancet, *2,271:1967.*

How the Little Guys Did It

Back in 1977, when the federal money tree seemed to be evergreen, the health bureaucracy announced a competition for EMS training grants. The idea was to fund the most worthy proposals for interdisciplinary training programs in emergency medical service. Many of the big medical schools submitted thick and fancy grant applications. Many of the country's regional EMS projects responded to the competition, for the most part applying the principle that grant applications are measured by the pound. And then there was the funny little application submitted by Durand-Vernon Ambulance (DVA), a volunteer service located about 20 miles southwest of Flint, Michigan.

DVA, like many volunteer EMS organizations, came to life when the town's funeral director quit the ambulance business. That was 14 years ago, but there are still several DVA members who remember when the organization's total assets consisted of a '63 Oldsmobile ambulance, a tank of gasoline and seven dollars. Not to mention the determination of DVA's founding members; they were *not* going to fail.

It was that determination to succeed which inspired the audacious grant application for federal training funds. When the idea was proposed to DVA members, few were confident that a little volunteer ambulance group from a little town of 4,000 could compete against the professional grantsmen and wordsmiths of America's most powerful educational and medical institutions. But they figured it wouldn't hurt to try.

The big guys were asking for big money. They wanted to hire project directors, curriculum specialists, clinical evaluators, coordinators of various types, and typists, receptionists and data clerks. Some of the big guys wanted money for brick and mortar — to build on to their existing educational castles. The bottom line figures ranged from a few hundred thousand to more than a million bucks.

The little guys from Durand, Michigan didn't want much. They needed some equipment to help train their members in basic life support, and to train the members of their community in CPR. They asked for about $10,000. Their application was approved and they got a little less than $8,000.

Federally funded programs come and go. A few years after the grants are announced, few people can remember what happened to the money or what it produced. We dropped by the headquarters of Durand-Vernon Ambulance last month. It's quite another story.

The training equipment has been in constant use since it was purchased nearly four years ago. Aside from helping the volunteers to improve their basic life support skills, several hundred residents of DVA's 167-square-mile service area have learned CPR on manikins supplied by the federal grant. Because most of DVA's volunteers are self-sufficient people who work with their hands, the equipment has been maintained in like-new condition.

Buoyed by their success in the national grant competition, DVA later responded to the ACT Foundation's 1978 offer of free CPR training manikins. The DVA proposal was clean, straightforward and honest. They demonstrated that they would make the most of a donated manikin. ACT forwarded the request to the National Automobile Dealers Association (NADA) Charitable Foundation with a recommendation for funding. The arrival of the NADA "Annie" in Durand was an occasion for a community celebration, and she has been in daily use ever since.

To our knowledge, the Durand-Vernon Ambulance organization is the only volunteer ambulance group in the United States ever to receive a federal training grant on its own. That grant did not make DVA exceptional; it was exceptional to begin with. But DVA proved that a little bit of federal money in the hands of the right people can produce as much as a lot of money in the hands of the professional grantees.

This very special group of men and women in this little town in mid-Michigan can serve as an example for volunteer organizations everywhere. Anything is possible. David can overcome Goliath. The volunteer ambulance service that concentrates on *service* won't have to worry about membership (DVA has a waiting list) or money (DVA has hired a business manager to watch over theirs).

If you're ever on the road between Lansing and Flint, I suggest you look for the little town of Durand. Stop in and get reacquainted with what America is all about. If you're lucky, the folks at DVA just might treat you to coffee and some of the best yellow cake you'll ever eat. They'll want you to inspect their array of training equipment, and the new training room they're building. We think you'll be as impressed as we were.

POSTSCRIPT: This appeared in JEMS *in 1981. One year later, Glenda Dolehanty, one of DVA's original members and its instructor-coordinator, was selected by the National Association of EMTs as EMT of the Year. In 1983, DVA was honored with the NAEMT's Leo R. Schwartz EMS Service of the Year award.*

A JEMS *staff member travels each year to the site of the "Best Service" to give a first-hand report to our readers. I eagerly returned in the early fall of 1983 for the assignment. There is a danger in being rated "The Best." It's easy to take the accolades too seriously. I saw no sign of that in Durand. Instead, I observed continuing emphasis on training and improvement. During my visit, a young member was wearing a T-shirt inscribed with the message: "I may be a volunteer, but I'm professional." It's more than a slogan in Durand, Michigan.*

Treasures in a Filing Cabinet

I'd reserved a Sunday afternoon to clean out some old files in my garage. Space had become a problem and the ultimate (but painful) task of throwing out some old treasures was upon me. I decided to get rid of everything dated 1975 or earlier. By day's end, I had thrown away nothing. Instead, I bought another filing cabinet and rearranged a bunch of stuff — and took an excursion across 10 years of EMS history. It was fun.

In 1975, EMS had an undisputed leader in David R. Boyd, MD, director of the division of EMS at the U.S. Department of HEW. He had blown into Washington the prior August and the dust didn't settle for seven years. In my garage are hundreds of items bearing witness to Boyd's years at the helm.

Before there was a federal EMS program, Dr. Dave Kluge of Rochester, N.Y., had created a national organization called STEP (Society for Total Emergency Programs). In 1975, I attended STEP's ninth annual conference in Indianapolis. The agenda and faculty list is stored in my garage. For a long time, Dave Kluge's STEP was the only organized voice for nationwide EMS improvements. But a voluntary group could not compete with the feds; the hoopla and federal bucks that Dave Boyd commanded were the swan song for STEP.

Another interesting event in '75 was the International Conference on Remote Emergency Medical Services at Texas Tech in Lubbock. The audience included Dave Boyd and other federal bureaucrats, a funeral home operator from Texas, physicians from about 10 states (as well as Montreal and Australia), folks from NASA and the military, a handful of EMTs and nurses, one nun and two lawyers. In those days, people came to conferences to find out what EMS was all about and whether they had a future in it. Most of those on the list in my garage were never again heard from.

In June '75, about 300 of us assembled in Washington for the First National Conference on Medical-Legal Implications of Emergency Medical Care. I dropped in while en route to a job interview in Buffalo. Dave Boyd was there, evangelizing for EMS and the federal program. Lots of hopeful grantees were there too, most of them posturing for a few minutes with the man whose funding decisions could make or break them.

I began 1975 in North Carolina and ended it as director of one of Dave Boyd's EMS projects — in Buffalo. In my garage are some wonderful recollections of those developmental days in EMS. Our eight-county project was based in a Regional Medical Program and our combined resources supported a staff of 13. We spent a lot of time in the field, selling the program, helping to upgrade local services, and generally carrying Boyd's message of "wall to wall" EMS in the U.S. We made lots of good friendships, many of which have endured over the years.

Dave Boyd's non-negotiable condition for getting refunded in '76 was to categorize hospitals in '75. With 400 miles between us and the nearest federal bureaucrat, with enough money and staff to get things done, my staff and I accepted that challenge. To my knowledge, we were the first to devise the "RFP" (request for proposals) scheme for designating specialty hospitals.

To underscore the categorization theme, Boyd held a national conference on that topic in Gerald Ford's hometown (Grand Rapids). It was a brash move but it got the President's attention. Most of us believed that the federal EMS program was as secure as national defense and would go on forever.

In my garage I found a ten-year-old issue of *JAMA* that contained Dr. Heimlich's description of his maneuver. In the same issue was an editorial by the medical establishment calling for the American Heart Association and others to collect and study data ". . . to determine the place of the Heimlich maneuver in the instruction of the public in proper emergency care practices." Did they ever settle that argument?*

In a folder all by itself I found one of my all-time favorite articles. In the July/August '75 issue of *JACEP*, Cleve Trimble and Roger Johnson helped us understand those who enter our EMS world with startling renditions of the "F" word. They wrote, "The singularly important lesson here is that no patient presents himself with the sole purpose of shouting four-letter Anglo-Saxon expletives in an attempt to shock female staff or to announce his aspiration for major political office." (*JACEP*, Vol. 4, No. 4)

Someday, when I am gone, my kids will have to dig

**See pp.47-56 — "Manuevering Around Heimlich."*

through my garage and get rid of all the jetsam and flotsam of their father's life. Till then, it will remain an undisturbed treasure trove of early EMS. After all, the only difference between a packrat and a librarian is the filing system.